BEYOND
DIET

BEYOND DIET

The 28-Day Metabolic
Breakthrough Plan

Martin Katahn, Ph.D.

Drawings by Patricia Sommers

W · W · Norton & Company · New York · London

Copyright © 1984 by Martin Katahn. All rights reserved. Published simultaneously in Canada by Stoddart, a subsidiary of General Publishing Co. Ltd, Don Mills, Ontario. Printed in the United States of America.

This book is composed in Baskerville. Composition and manufacturing by The Haddon Craftsmen.

Library of Congress Cataloging in Publication Data
Katahn, Martin.
  Beyond diet, the 28-day metabolic breakthrough plan.
  Bibliography: p
  Includes index.
  1. Reducing diets. 2. Metabolism. I. Title
RM222.2.K346 1984   613.2'5   83-25029

ISBN 0-393-01852-0

W. W. Norton & Company, Inc., 500 Fifth Avenue, New York, N. Y. 10110
W. W. Norton & Company Ltd., 37 Great Russell Street, London WC1B 3NU

5 6 7 8 9 0

To Enid, Terri, and
David, Who Make It
All Possible

CONTENTS

8 / Contents

III
Your Fat-Burning Insurance Policy

IV
The Scientific Background

V
The Psychology of Successful Weight Management

VI

The Great Escape, or Are You a Refugee from a Low-Calorie Diet?

ACKNOWLEDGMENTS

Many persons have played a significant role in helping me write this book.

I am indebted to my colleagues and co-directors of the Vanderbilt Weight Management Program, Drs. John Pleas and Kenneth Wallston, with whose help the concepts that underly the Metabolic Breakthrough Plan were developed and tested. One of my former graduate students, Dr. Mark McMinn, contributed greatly to the research on the biochemical aspects of obesity.

In its actual writing, this book was a family affair. Without the help of my wife, Enid, my daughter, Terri, and my son, David, it would have been far more difficult to complete. All of us have spent many hours in the kitchen working to apply the principles of food preparation that I present in this book to various styles of cooking from around the world. Special thanks to Terri for being so helpful when we had writing deadlines to meet during the revision stages.

Once again I want to thank my editor at W.W. Norton, Starling Lawrence, whose astute comments have helped me improve the clarity of presentation, and my agents, Arthur and Richard Pine, who, together with Star, have given me so much support and encouragement.

And finally, there's that marvelous machine, my TRS80 computer and word processor. It has never been sick, nor has it taken a vacation in the year and a half that I have used it for writing and data processing. It performs without complaint from dawn 'til dusk, and thereafter as needed. Many thanks to my friends at Radio Shack for making this tremendous technological advance possible, for helping me learn to use it so efficiently, and for making sure that I never lost a single day of work during this entire period of time.

PART I

The 28-Day Metabolic Breakthrough Plan: What Is It and What's in It for You?

1

THROWING AWAY YOUR DIET

Do you count yourself among those millions of persons who have lost weight innumerable times on one of the popular low-calorie diets, only to put it all back on again time after time?

Have you heard of a brand new quick weight-loss program and are you thinking of beginning another diet?

Please take my advice—Don't!

Don't start on that diet until you read what I have to say. You may change your mind.

You may already have a "fat" metabolism, and that low-calorie diet is only going to make it worse!

There are no ifs, ands, or buts about it.

Let me give you a brief explanation for starters. There's a good deal more to come.

That word "metabolism" refers to all the things your body does to change the nutrients in food into the form your body needs to stay alive.

Right now I'm concerned with the energy part—the calories in your food.

Some people have stingy, or "fat," metabolisms. From the moment digestion begins, everything is done with as little wasted energy as possible. When you have one of these miserly, "fat" metabolisms, your body does its work so efficiently that, in comparison with the average person, there are many more calories left over to be put into your "fat banks" for storage.

You can be born with a "fat" metabolism, but what's really worse is that *you can eat and act in a way that changes a perfectly normal, or "thin," metabolism into a "fat" one!*

Here are just a few of the facts that I am going to explain, which you need to understand if you are finally going to be successful in your pursuit of health, fitness, and desirable weight:

1. Most people who are overweight do, indeed, have at least a slight genetically determined predisposition to accumulate more than the average amount of body fat.

2. But it is only a *predisposition.* All people, even those with inherited tendencies to overweight, can make a significant impact on their metabolic processes. You can cultivate a "thin" metabolism.

3. Dieting as a means of weight control can *increase* your fat-storage capacity. It simply makes your body even more stingy with calories. When you finish each and every low-calorie diet you can end up gaining weight by *eating less* than you did before you began your diet in the first place.

4. *When you eat,*
   how often you eat,
   as well as what you eat
all make a difference in your metabolism.

Two people can be eating the same total number of calories each day, but one may be considerably fatter than the other if that person, without fully understanding the process, has fallen into a fat way of eating while the other has cultivated a thin style of eating.

5. A modest change in physical activity can *guarantee that you will NEVER regain any weight you lose* when you follow the 28-day plan that I will give you to reach desirable weight.

6. But not all activity provides equal benefit.
   What you do,
   when you do it,
   as well as how much you do
all make some activities worth more in terms of metabolic improvement and weight control than others.

Beyond Diet contains a total metabolism improvement program that shows you how to make a *breakthrough* in your metabolic processes. It helps you put into practice the unique combination of scientifically proven principles for weight loss and permanent weight maintenance that my colleagues and I have developed after seven years' research into over two thousand weight-loss cases in the Vanderbilt University Weight Management Program.

I have put these principles to the test with some of the most difficult weight-loss problems—people who have tried every diet available, from Scarsdale to Beverly Hills and back, with stopovers on total fasts and protein powders in between, only to regain whatever they lost and then some.

Why didn't these diets work?

It wasn't because these folks weren't trying!

I don't have to tell you—overweight persons are always trying. In fact, according to the intake dietary histories of persons entering the Vanderbilt program, overweight people go on an average of two formal diets a year, in addition to other short-term efforts to restrain their eating.

Here are just a few of the reasons why this pattern of dieting only makes weight control more difficult (fuller explanations are given later in the book):

1. Repeated dieting can make your gut get *larger,* NOT smaller.

2. After using such low-calorie diets, a whole bunch of enzymes that help digest food in your intestines get abnormally active. Ordinarily, a certain percentage of the calories in food is not digested, but, after such diets, these enzymes work extra hard to extract every single one.

3. Your "fat" metabolism really turns on after a low-calorie diet. As the calories from your food enter your bloodstream, your switched-on miserly metabolism doesn't burn them at a normal rate. It may take only 60 calories to do the work that formerly took 100. This keeps you locked into continuous dieting, because, if you return to your pre-diet intake, your "fat" metabolism can push 40 calories out of every 100 into fat storage.

4. Compared with before the diet, certain enzymes in your fat cells increase in activity and take up any fat you have eaten faster than ever. I guess that should not come as a surprise to you—every dieter knows that it's easier to fill up fat cells after a diet than to empty them when you're trying to lose weight.

Perhaps you can see the ultimate outcome: instead of making it easier to get thin and stay that way, low-calorie diets can take a "fat" metabolism and make it fatter. And, if you have just begun to put on weight for the first time in your life, the use of a low-calorie diet can actually change a normal metabolism into a "fat" one.

In the 28-Day Metabolic Breakthrough Plan I will give you an alternative to this unhappy situation.

If you put these Breakthrough principles to work, as our former dieters do when they finish the Vanderbilt program, you can end up six months down the line 50 pounds lighter. Within just 28 days, however, you will be doing *exactly* what it takes to keep those 50 pounds of fat off your body forever. You've got 75 to lose? That's no problem either. Of course, you can't lose 75 pounds in 28 days, but the goal of the Metabolic Breakthrough Plan is to reprogram your metabolic processes to burn calories rather than store them, as it presently does, and in just 28 days you will have put that program into action. From that point on, you can be absolutely confident that, once you reach your desired weight, you will be able to return to eating the same amount you do today, and never regain a pound.

I know that this sounds too good to be true. So, all I can say to you at this point is: read the rationale and begin your own 28-Day Breakthrough Program. Your day-by-day guide begins on page 85. Then, as your weight comes off, you may wish to study the later chapters in which I present, in greater detail, the physiological and biochemical bases on which the program is founded.

Because there are so many people who have used diets of 800 or fewer calories in the recent past, I have written a special section (Chapters 26 and 27) to help people get back to normal after such diets, or to continue losing weight when necessary.

If you have just finished one of these low-calorie diets, have reached ideal weight, and are *happy* with your maintenance plan, I think that's marvelous and I hope you are eating nutritiously. However, in case you would like to be more relaxed about your maintenance program and *want the freedom to add several hundred calories a day* to your eating plan, I'll show you how to do it with some special modifications to the 28-Day Breakthrough Plan.

If you have achieved only part of your goal or have started to regain weight after any low-calorie diet, I will show you how to get back on track and achieve the success that has eluded you or, in the latter case, how to nip this unfortunate process in the bud.

Let's not turn victory, or near-victory, into defeat!

Throughout the book I will refer to case histories and research from laboratories all around the world, as well as from our own research at Vanderbilt. I also will present data gathered from my own experience with different diets.

I have experimented with a number of the popular approaches

—the "fad" diets—so as to determine their effects on my own body and to verify the reports of people who have used such diets. In addition, I wanted to see if the startling effects that are obtained in research with animals on low-calorie diets could be replicated in myself so that I could be more certain that the research could be generalized to other human beings.

But my research in the area of obesity is only part of the story. In addition to my work as director of the Vanderbilt University Weight Management Program, I have had personal experience with the very real problem of being severely overweight.

Twenty years ago, at the age of thirty-five, I weighed 75 pounds more than I do today. I suffered from hypertension and had a heart problem to go along with those extra pounds. The following question was really put to me: just how much did I want to live to see my children grow up and enjoy the company of that very special woman who is my wife?

I lost that weight by happily stumbling across the principles that lead to permanent weight control, without having any conscious idea that twenty years later these principles would find a foundation in solid scientific research. Today, at fifty-five years of age, I *must* eat almost 3000 calories a day just to maintain myself at my ideal weight of 154 pounds (5 feet 10½ inches tall). I can eat more today than I ever could as a fat man, and my daily intake is about 600 calories higher than the average male as much as twenty years younger than I am.

And my exercise cardiogram, which twenty years ago might have suggested a bypass operation, now looks perfectly normal.

My goal in *Beyond Diet* is to put you, within 28 days, on the road to a permanent metabolic improvement that will enable you to eat like a normal human being without dieting, just as I do and just as those successful persons do whose experiences I am going to relate.

You can read this book with the assurance that, as a responsible health professional and a former fat man, I am presenting this program with your total health and welfare first and foremost in my mind.

I have no product to sell—no vitamins, no powdered formula foods, and no miraculous pills with secret ingredients.

I run no weight-loss clinic for profit—all funds generated by our program are used for research.

My primary objective in writing this book is to tell you everything

I know about the problem of obesity, and everything I know that will enable you to make your own metabolic breakthrough. When you follow the 28-Day Plan, it means losing weight and keeping it off forever.

If you try it, I think you will like it. It's a lot more fun than being fat, and it works much, much better than dieting.

You can see the effects for yourself in just 28 days, and then you, too, can be another living proof.

2

METABOLISM: SLOWING DOWN
OR REVVING UP

"I have about 50 pounds to lose. Why shouldn't I just choose a low-calorie diet program, or one of those powdered formula diets, and get it off as quickly as possible?"

If you have a difficult weight problem, you may have been simply aggravating it, if not actually creating it, if you have ever used the kind of diet you're asking about. Such diets—anything under 800 calories a day, and possibly anything under 1000 calories a day—can alter your metabolism.[1,2] They slow it down. When you go on a low-calorie diet, you give your body practice on how to "eat less, and weigh more."[3]

I have the data to prove this to you. I also have the data to show you that it needn't be this way, if you will follow the principles of the 28-Day Metabolic Breakthrough Plan.

Before me on my desk is a stack of daily eating and activity records, a pile of case histories, and files filled with descriptions of various weight-control programs. They clearly illustrate the amazing power we have over our bodies to either increase or decrease our daily metabolic needs.

In particular, I want to tell you what I see in the written daily eating records that have been kept for me, for research purposes, by people who have lost weight on one of the quick-loss, low-calorie formula diets. I want to contrast these records, which were obtained during the first few months following their weight loss, with those of other persons who have followed the suggestions I am going to

---

[1]Superscripts refer to References placed by chapter at the back of the book.

make to you—and who have kept huge amounts of weight off not for just a few months but for at least five years after participating in the Vanderbilt program.

The women who lost weight on the powdered formula diet are now eating an average of approximately 1250 calories a day (including one or two packages of their formula). While that number of calories is about one-third less than the needs of the average American woman as estimated by the Food and Nutrition Board of the National Research Council, *if these women eat any more than that, they will start to gain weight.*

The eating and activity records of the women who are following the suggestions I am going to make to you in the 28-Day Metabolic Breakthrough Plan offer a happy contrast. *They are eating over 1900 calories a day and they are not regaining any of the weight they have lost.*

The contrast in the records of the men using both approaches is just as striking. After using the formula diet, the men average about 1600 to 1800 calories per day to maintain their weight. The record of one of the men is especially informative. He used the record-keeping task as a motivation to *try* to lose a little more weight. I say "try" because, averaging 1350 calories per day during the week of record keeping, *he didn't lose a pound!*

The men who now follow the suggestions I will make to you are averaging over 2700 calories per day. They are not regaining any of the weight they lost over five years ago.*

How can this be?

Were these people different to begin with, or have they, with their eating and activity behavior, either slowed down or "revved up" their metabolic processes?

Before I can give you an understandable answer to that question, I need to explain some important facts about metabolism.

You and Your Metabolism

Although we often refer to our "metabolism" with a sense of mystery and feelings of frustration, especially if we think it's on the slow side and fighting our weight-loss efforts, only recently have health professionals begun to understand the full importance of

*This research was first reported in an address to the New York Academy of Science, November 5, 1982, and is in press as *Annals* of the Academy.[4]

metabolic variability, and to appreciate the effect that our eating and activity habits can have on our metabolic processes.

To begin with, the word *metabolism* refers to all of the biochemical processes through which the food you eat is broken down and its nutritional components transformed for use in rebuilding tissue, constructing your various hormones and enzymes, and supplying the energy you need to move your body and keep your vital functions going.

Some people have what biochemists call "thrifty," or very efficient, metabolisms; others have wasteful, or inefficient, metabolisms. You can be born with tendencies one way or the other (see Chapter 19 for a full discussion) and you can change from one to another, according to your eating and activity behaviors.

When it comes to metabolic improvement for overweight people, you want to go from thrifty to wasteful, from being very efficient in the way you use food energy to being very inefficient.

Let me give you an example to illustrate, by analogy, what I mean.

Think of some persons you know who are very inefficient—they make many trips to get a simple job done—and they are constantly active even when it's not necessary. Even when sitting still, carrying on a conversation, they cross and uncross their legs, tap their fingers, and use their hands and arms to express themselves—all unnecessary actions when it comes to having a conversation.

Then think of some persons who are the exact opposite—always perfectly organized, no wasted motion, no extra trips; when they settle down for a pleasant conversation, they really know how to relax.

Now, apply this analogy down to the cellular level of your body. You have literally billions upon billions of nerve cells, muscle cells, fat cells, blood cells, and many other kinds of cells. Right down at the cellular level of your body, these cells can behave like the first group of persons I described, and use up a lot of energy just spinning their wheels as they get their jobs done. This wastefulness can actually be measured in the laboratory, because wasteful cells give off more heat as they do their work compared with efficient cells.[5] *Naturally thin people have inefficient, wasteful cells.*

Naturally fat people have those thrifty, or efficient, cells. This means that, after the energy from food is made available for bodily processes, there is an extra amount left over to be put into their fat cells for storage. Having this "thrifty trait" is great when we are faced with an uncertain food supply, and it assured the survival of the human race in times past. But it certainly doesn't work to our advantage when we have plenty of high-fat and processed foods to eat, and machines to do the work that might otherwise burn up a larger portion of our daily calories.

When I speak of metabolic improvement for overweight people, I'm talking about the things you can do, with surprisingly simple changes in the way you eat and in your activity level, to turn your thrifty metabolic system into the most extravagant user of energy that is humanly possible, given your genetic heritage. Contrary to what seems to be ordinary common sense, the more wasteful you get, the better.

And now let me return to that question I asked earlier on page 22 and phrase it in a way that is pertinent to your own weight problem:

"Can you, with your own eating and activity behaviors, influence your hereditary, metabolic predisposition toward obesity?"

The answer is, emphatically, "Yes!"

If you attempt to control your weight with low-calorie diets, however, you can change an already "thrifty" metabolism into a very, VERY thrifty metabolism and perhaps never again be able to eat like a normal human being. I explain this more fully in the next chapter.

But if you follow my suggestions, I can guarantee you a much more felicitous outcome. Even if you are 50 or 75 pounds overweight, as I was twenty years ago, there is every likelihood that you can eat the same total number of calories you do today and never regain a pound after you reach your desired weight.

You can make one or more changes in the number of meals you eat, the size of the meals, the time of day when you eat, and the particular nutrient composition of those meals. Because your body is such a marvelous, adaptive organism that learns from experience (just think of all the things you've learned in your lifetime), these changes in your behavior actually "teach" it to waste 10 to 20 percent of the energy content of your daily diet. And, by the way, this style of eating is the healthiest and most natural way known to man.

Then, with some modest changes in your activity level, you will be programming your body to burn enough additional calories so that you will be able to add another 10 to 20 percent to your total daily calorie requirements.

There may, in fact, be an even more ideal final outcome awaiting you at the end of your Metabolic Breakthrough Plan: you may discover that you will be able to eat *more* at your ideal weight than you ever ate as a fat person.

3

THE CASE AGAINST LOW-CALORIE DIETS

You know it in your bones, as well as in your fat cells:
DIETS DON'T WORK!

The reason that diets have so little chance of success is that they slow what may be an already thrifty metabolism even further, which translates into a continuous need for further dieting. It can become a vicious cycle, which works in the following way:

Your body has a wisdom of its own built into it as a result of some two million years of evolution during which time mankind—and what's even more important to the problem of obesity, *in which womankind*—faced periodic famines. Today, living as we do in our affluent Western world, feeling confident of a dependable food supply, it is hard for us to appreciate that about 70 percent of the world's population faces a food shortage once every two years, and about 25 percent of the world's population experiences such shortages twice a year.

When you go on a low-calorie diet, your body doesn't understand your wish to look better and feel better; it thinks you are about to starve it to death. And, in that wisdom built into your genes as a result of our evolutionary heritage, your body cuts back on its metabolic needs by as much as 35 or even 45 percent.[1,2]

The female body seems to be better at achieving this metabolic cutback than the male body. It's only logical that nature should have worked it out this way, considering the fact that women have their own special responsibility for seeing to it that the human race survives in times of famine. After all, it is the female of the species that

carries the unborn young and, historically, had the full responsibility of nourishing the newborn for many months after birth. It takes
from 40,000 to 80,000 extra calories to carry a baby for nine
months, and about 850 extra calories per day to nurse it. The ability
to store more fat to begin with, to increase fat during pregnancy,
and to resist famine (read "diets") is nature's way of meeting this
responsibility for the survival of the species in the female body.

This inborn ability to resist diets is illustrated in Figure 3-1.

When you first begin a low-calorie diet, everything seems just
great. Weight seems to be pouring off (it is, in fact, "pouring off,"
but pouring off water, not fat). Within three weeks after you begin

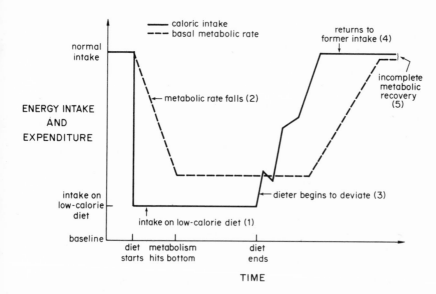

FIGURE 3-1.   Metabolic reactions to a low-calorie diet. Person
desiring to lose weight cuts calories dramatically (1). Metabolic rate
begins to slow and hits bottom in three to seven weeks (2). There is
now little discrepancy between intake and lowered metabolic needs.
Dieter gets discouraged and begins to deviate (3). Dieter "half-diets"
for a time, but soon returns to former intake (4). However, weight
gain will now occur on fewer calories than it previously took to maintain a higher weight. Metabolic processes may not return to normal
or near-normal for an extended period of time (5). Dieter ends up
heavier than before starting to diet.

a low-calorie diet, however, you will have dehydrated yourself as far as you can and your body's energy needs will have dropped to the point where you can hit frequent plateaus and experience hardly any weight loss.

Then, the moment you get discouraged and deviate in the slightest degree, what do you get? A quick weight gain that can equal 3 pounds overnight, even though you may have eaten only a single cup of onion soup, which happens to be high in sodium, or only one sweet potato and two chocolate-chip cookies. (We have verified these weight gains as a result of such additions to a diet in the Vanderbilt program.)

And then what happens? If you keep on with only slight deviations from your diet—"half-dieting," as it were—you will start to gain weight on fewer calories than it took for you to maintain your weight before you ever started your diet in the first place.

Of course, your metabolic rate turns back on again and starts to rise as you begin to eat more, *but it may not return to near normal until you have regained a good part of the weight you have lost.* There is even some chance that, if you have severely curtailed your intake and don't take special steps to elevate your metabolism, your metabolic rate may remain below your pre-diet level for a considerable time thereafter. If you eat again exactly at your pre-diet level, you will end up gaining several additional pounds. Thus, if you weighed 200 pounds before your diet, when you resume your regular eating habits, this lowered metabolic rate will cause you to accumulate an extra 10 pounds—so that you will weigh 210 pounds—even though your food intake is the same as before your diet.

If you decide to diet again in another effort to control your weight, your body may turn down its metabolic activity faster than it did the time before. Your previous diet gave it practice in conservation. It's a simple process of adaptation: if you keep on giving your body practice in getting along on less food, it learns to do it better and better. Mother Nature isn't dumb—we are![3,4]

Given this situation, is it any wonder that the weight curve of the continually dieting adult looks something like an ascending staircase, going ever higher after a temporary diet-induced dip or valley?

But this is only part of the story.

Once you start to eat again after a low-calorie diet, your fat cells spring into action, pulling the calories right out of the bloodstream faster than ever before. The enzyme responsible—called adipose tissue lipoprotein lipase (AT-LPL)—can become three, four, or even several times more energetic in its fat-storage activity after a diet than before. In one study, AT-LPL activity did not return to near normal in volunteers who had been on a 600-calorie diet until their body weights had risen to 105 percent of their original pre-diet levels.[5]

All of the research on the effects of low-calorie dieting adds up to one indisputable fact: When you finish using a low-calorie diet, you may not be able to eat more than about 60 percent of your pre-diet intake without gaining weight!

This has been demonstrated in research with animals,[6] and I have demonstrated the effects in myself. And, by researching the maintenance plans of those quick weight-loss programs whose enticing advertisements you can read in your daily papers, I have found that, after you finish using such low-calorie approaches to weight loss, you may be obliged to stick with about 1200 calories per day if you are a woman, 1600 to 1800 if you are a man, for an indefinite period. *Otherwise you will gain weight.*

If you doubt my word, have an interview at any of these programs that puts you on a diet of 800 calories or less. Ask to see the "lifetime" maintenance plan. You will find that these maintenance plans call for caloric intakes between 30 and 40 percent below the averages suggested by the National Research Council.

This leads me to suggest that, if you are ever tempted to use such low-calorie diets, you ought to try out the recommended maintenance plan *first.* Before you pay out a penny, get on that maintenance plan for a month or two. See if you care to live with it for the rest of your life! If you can't live with the maintenance plan, what's the use of suffering their diet when the ultimate outcome will see you weighing several pounds more than ever before?

A Personal Experiment

In the summer of 1981 I performed a study using the Beverly Hills Diet as a result of an article in which its creator, Ms. Judy Mazel, claimed that the diet was safe for runners. The outcome was exactly the same as when I experimented with the Scarsdale Diet two years earlier. As you may recall, the Beverly Hills Diet calls for fruit only during the first 10 days, whereas the Scarsdale Diet is a high-protein diet.

Using the Beverly Hills Diet on this occasion, and stuffing myself with as much fruit as I could tolerate, my intake was approximately 1100 calories per day.

I lost nine pounds in one week, while maintaining my usual level of physical activity. I experienced a variety of symptoms that frequently accompany all low-calorie diets no matter how they combine the proportions of protein and carbohydrate. These symptoms included an elevation in heart rate of 30 percent on a standard fitness test (jogging at a pace of a mile in ten minutes) which resulted from a decrease in blood volume (hypovolemia). With low blood volume, your heart must work harder and beat faster to get sufficient oxygen to exercising muscles.

You don't have to be doing anything special in the way of physical activity, however, to experience the effects of low blood volume when you are on a low-calorie diet: even in a sedentary person, it leads to dizziness when you get up quickly from a sitting or prone position (orthostatic hypotension). In addition, low blood volume decreases the body's ability to cool itself in hot weather. This can make a person more susceptible to heat exhaustion or possibly heat stroke. There simply isn't enough blood getting to the surface of the skin to keep the body cool. If you do exercise under these conditions, you must be very careful, as I discovered when I used the Scarsdale Diet: on the fifth day, after losing 5 pounds, I almost fainted trying to complete a tennis match in 90-degree heat.

In the third day of the Beverly Hills Diet, I began awakening in the middle of the night with a slight trembling feeling. This continued to the end of the week.

Now, I am experienced in monitoring myself and can prevent serious consequences when I experiment with different diets while maintaining my customary high level of physical activity. But, all of the symptoms I have just mentioned are signs of a pre-shock syndrome.

So, naturally, I stopped using the Beverly Hills Diet after one week.

One of my reasons for investigating this last diet, however, was to determine what would happen *after* using it. Of great importance to the argument I make against low-calorie diets is the fact that I could not eat more than 66 percent of my pre-diet intake without gaining weight for the next three weeks. This occurred in spite of my usual level of physical activity, which involves between 35 and 40 miles a week of jogging and an occasional tennis match. (I know that this calorie count is accurate because I weigh and measure every bite of food when I do experiments of this nature.)

After three weeks of feeling lousy and looking pretty bad while I was restricting myself to approximately 2000 calories a day (my colleagues all thought I was ill), I felt I had proved my point and resumed my normal food intake, which is almost 3000 calories per day.

I will present additional laboratory findings on the effects of low-calorie dieting when I go more deeply into the physiological basis of obesity in Chapter 20.

Right now I am eager to move on quickly, help you determine how your present eating habits affect your metabolic functions, and get you started on your way to permanent control of your weight.

You can rest assured that when you go beyond diet into the 28-Day Metabolic Breakthrough Plan you will not suffer any of the side effects of low-calorie dieting and you will end up at your desired weight able to eat about 30 to 40 percent more food than when you finish one of the low-calorie approaches.

4

DO YOU HAVE A FAT STYLE OF EATING?

It may not be how much you eat, but when, what, and how often that are forcing your metabolism into thrifty habits and helping you stay fat.

The research on this matter is quite convincing: of thirteen studies that have compared the *total* caloric intake of overweight with average-weight persons, six show no difference, five show that the overweight individuals eat *less* than average, and only two show that they eat more.[1]

Nevertheless, there really is such a thing as a "fat style of eating" and you may have it. You may in truth be eating no more than your friends who weigh 40 or 50 pounds less than you do, but you may be eating in such a way as to convert 10 or even 20 percent of your intake to fat unnecessarily!

Here is a short Eating Habits Test that will determine whether or not you have a fat style of eating (there is another Eating Habits Test on p. 249, which focuses on the psychological and environmental factors associated with being overweight).

1. Do you eat most of your food in one large meal each day?
2. Is that one large meal at night?
3. Does your food intake vary drastically from day to day (e.g., big weekends followed by several days of restrained eating)?
4. Do you go without food for a full twenty-four hours on a frequent basis?
5. Do you use a low-calorie diet periodically (one or more times a year) for more than a week at a time?

6. Do you tend to eat more processed foods (snacks, white bread, refined cereals) than you do whole grains (whole-wheat breads and cereals, rice, etc.)?

7. Do you eat more high-fat and sugar foods (fried food, desserts, candy, soft drinks), or alcohol, than you do fresh fruits and vegetables?

8. Do you eat fewer than eight servings of foods from the whole-grain, legume, fruit, and vegetable categories each day?

A single "yes" answer to any one of these questions can mean that you have a fat style of eating. Your style of eating unnecessarily maximizes the conversion of the calories in your food to fat.

But, you say, "A calorie is a calorie. Aren't all calories the same?"

Of course they are—in the laboratory.

A calorie is simply a measure of the energy content of food. It's the amount of energy necessary to raise the temperature of 1 kilogram of water 1 degree Celsius. It doesn't matter whether that calorie comes from fat, carbohydrate, or protein, and it doesn't matter what time of day you measure it—in the laboratory, that is.

But it does matter to the human body.

The human body processes food differently depending upon when you eat it, how frequently you eat, how much food is in a given meal, how much fiber it contains, and whether there happens to be a surplus of fat in your diet rather than carbohydrate or protein relative to your immediate caloric needs.

Here are some very important facts for overweight people:

1. Animals that are permitted to eat for only two hours per day, rather than freely, according to their natural inclinations, end up 30 percent heavier than normal.[2]

2. Animals that are intermittently fasted (e.g., 2 days per week) show an increased ability to convert food to fat and a higher percentage of their body weight turns to fat.[3]

3. Animals fed according to the patterns just described show an *increase* in the size and weight of the stomach and small intestines.[3] In other words, contrary to popular belief, dieting does *not* reduce the size of the stomach.

4. Each time you eat, the body revs up in order to digest your food and your metabolic rate increases. But not all of the energy taken from your food is put to work maintaining essential processes. A good deal of it is simply wasted, and given off as heat. The energy

that is "wasted" after meals is called the *thermic effect of food.*

The thermic effect is greatest after breakfast, when you may waste up to 10 percent of the calories you take in at that meal. It is likely to be less at lunch, and lower yet at dinner.[4]

5. If you go on a low-calorie diet, your body eliminates all or part of this thermic effect in an effort to conserve energy and maintain your weight.

6. You may waste more of the calories in your food, and convert fewer of them to fat storage between meals, if you eat many small meals each day, rather than a couple of larger ones. While it is not entirely clear what leads to what, people who eat five or more times per day are slimmer than those who eat three or fewer meals.[3]

7. People who eat a high-fiber diet (foods from the complex carbohydrate category in general—whole grains, fruits, vegetables, and legumes) have greater intestinal motility. Food goes through their systems more quickly and more smoothly. In addition, according to a United States Department of Agriculture report, the fiber combines with a certain proportion of the fat present in the diet and prevents it from being absorbed. If you have at least two servings of a high-fiber food with each meal, and eat high-fiber snacks, you will prevent 10 percent or more of your total fat intake from being absorbed.

8. It is easier to get fat on a high-fat diet than on a diet in which surplus calories come from protein or carbohydrates. Your metabolism uses four or five times more energy to convert protein and carbohydrates for storage in your fat cells than it uses to convert dietary fat for fat storage.

For example, consider a large evening meal of around 1000 calories, capping off a day of relatively little physical activity. If 500 of these calories are derived from fat, 475 of them can end up in your fat cells since it only takes about 5 percent of the energy in the fat to make the necessary conversion. If you substituted 500 calories of carbohydrate, only about 400 of them could find their way ultimately into your fat cells since it takes about 20 percent of the energy available in the carbohydrate to convert it for fat storage.[5] When you consider that this process may be repeated daily after a large evening meal with a high fat content, the importance of deriving more of your calories from complex carbohydrates and low-fat sources of protein becomes obvious.

You now have the facts.

If you answered even one of the questions in the Eating Habits Test in the "fat style of eating" direction, you can easily be eating your way to obesity without eating any more calories than the "naturally" thin person who has perhaps unconsciously, but fortunately, cultivated a "slim" style of eating.

Are you ready to make a few changes?

5

EATING SLIM

If your answers on the Eating Habits Test in the last chapter tell
you that you have an eating style that contributes to your weight
problem, you can make a significant difference with one or two small
changes.

Don't think you must aim for perfection, however. Each change,
no matter how small, can make a difference.

Here is a summary of the general principles that can reprogram
your metabolic processes and permit you to eat more and weigh
less.

1. Eat many smaller meals each day, rather than one or two large
ones.

2. Eat as much as you can earlier in the day, rather than later.
Eating 50 to 60 percent of your food intake before 1:00 P.M. will be
an improvement if you have been skipping breakfast, and 75 percent
will be ideal.*

3. Avoid drastic variation in your intake from day to day as much
as possible; especially avoid skipping food for periods of twenty-
four hours at a time on any regular basis. (Of course, if you have
overeaten it is better to take immediate remedial action and cut back
slightly rather than to wait until the situation gets completely out of
hand. But, a regular rotation of feasts and famines makes weight
control more difficult.)

4. Avoid low-calorie diets and, if you are a sedentary person,

---

*Not much is known about the metabolic variations in people who keep irregular
hours, but some of the hormone and enzyme rhythms do change under these conditions. If you have an unusual schedule, I would simply advise switching more of your
intake to the first five or six hours of your day.

never diet without simultaneously increasing your physical activity.

5. Reduce the amount of fat in your diet and increase your consumption of whole grains, fresh fruits, and vegetables.

6. Have two servings of high-fiber foods with each meal and get in the habit of eating high-fiber snacks.

Some of these changes are easier to make than others, and some are more important than others. Fortunately, the most important alterations from a metabolic improvement standpoint are the easiest, rather than the hardest, to make.

The two most important changes you can make are to avoid low-calorie diets (that's not going to be hard, is it?) and to decrease foods that are high in fat or otherwise "dense in calories" in comparison with their other nutrient content of vitamins, minerals, and dietary fiber. Unfortunately, reducing fats and increasing fruits, vegetables, and whole grains is a little harder for most people to accomplish than avoiding low-calorie diets. So, for this reason, I have developed the AC/DC ratio, which is a shortcut formula for sound nutrition and which simultaneously ensures that you will obtain the metabolic benefits of a high-fiber, low-fat diet.

6

THE AC/DC FORMULA: THE KEY
TO SOUND NUTRITION

The single most important change you can make in your diet is to *A*ccent complex *C*arbohydrates and use them to substitute as often as you can for foods *D*ense in *C*alories. This leads to what I call, for short, the AC/DC formula, or AC/DC ratio.

In the lists of foods that follow, a ratio of 8 to 2, that is, a choice of eight servings of foods from the AC list and two allowances from the DC list, is the ideal AC/DC ratio for sound nutrition and successful weight management.*

Why and how does it work?

It works because, first and foremost, AC foods in general contain large amounts of fiber, and *fiber is a fat blocker.* When you have two servings of foods from the AC list with each meal, and use them as between-meal snacks, 10 percent and possibly more of the fat calories in your diet get tangled up in the roughage and never get digested. If they can't get digested, they can't end up in the cozy confines of your fat cells.

Think of what this means in terms of weight control. Have you been gaining weight at the rate of 10, or even 20, pounds a year? If you had incorporated the ideal, 8 to 2 AC/DC ratio in your diet, this might never have happened. Would you like to see that weight

---

*The AC/DC ratio is, of course, associated with an adequate intake of calcium and protein from the Milk and Meat food groups, or from suitable substitutes. The complete Metabolic Breakthrough Nutrition Plan is presented in Chapter 14. I am focusing here on the key aspect of the plan that will do the most to facilitate weight loss and permanent weight management.

vanish without cutting calories and never return? Just switch to the AC/DC ratio, and it will happen naturally, without "dieting." Combine it with one or two of my other suggestions, and you can be a *permanent 50 pounds lighter within six months.*

The substitution of AC foods for DC foods can have a profound effect on your metabolic processes. In a study presented at the International Congress on Obesity held in New York in October 1983, Dr. S. H. Blondheim of the Hebrew University–Hadassah Medical School in Jerusalem reported that the consumption of equivalent calories from foods in the AC category (such as fruits), compared with foods in the DC category (such as a candy bar), will cause an increase in the metabolic rate *six times greater.* While one serving of a DC food, such as a chocolate bar, might cause a 1 to 2 percent elevation in metabolic rate, fruits and vegetables containing the same number of calories can cause it to rise almost 10 percent. This is the thermic effect of food I have already mentioned in Chapter 4 and discuss more fully in Chapter 19. In other words, high-fiber foods can cause your system to rev up and burn more calories during the digestive process than do dense-calorie foods.

The AC/DC formula works for yet another reason. AC foods are high in bulk and fill you up more quickly than foods that have many calories and little fiber. When you eat balanced meals that contain a variety of nutrients, the fat and protein in your meal will stay in your stomach longer and provide the long-lasting feeling of satiety after the bulk has given you the "full" feeling. But, remember, not as much of the fat will actually get digested when the meal has had plenty of fiber.

You obtain several other health benefits by adhering to the AC/DC formula. The fiber in complex carbohydrates seems to lower blood glucose levels and reduce insulin requirements in the case of diabetes. Fiber may also have positive effects on plasma lipids and cholesterol.[1] In addition, as you increase fiber, you will tend to increase your intake of vitamins A and C. All three of these nutrients, which tend to be on the low side in the typical American diet, have been shown to prevent certain forms of cancer.

When you switch to the AC/DC formula, you don't really "go on a diet." You can still eat some of those DC foods—the cakes, cookies, other desserts, and your favorite salad dressings—but, for quick results, you make sure you get those eight servings of high-fiber foods from the AC list and never go over two allowances from the DC list until you see whether you are losing weight at a satisfactory rate. Get in the mood to substitute an AC food for foods on the DC list, until you reach that total of eight servings per day. Use fruits for snacks. They will make it easy to reach the ideal total.

Although no calorie-counting and no eating diaries are required when you implement the AC/DC formula and begin the Metabolic Breakthrough Plan, many people do find that keeping a simple count of the number of AC foods they have had each day is helpful. If you vow to reach your total of eight servings from the AC list *before* you have that second DC allowance, you can't fail.

Keep a simple tally on a scrap of paper each day, or in a pocket-sized notebook. Each time you choose a serving of food from the AC list, just write down the letter "A." When you choose a DC food, write a "D."

An even easier tally can be kept by making a little mark with a pencil, or felt-tipped pen, on the back of your left hand whenever you make an AC choice. Make a mark on the back of your right hand for each DC allowance. Never make more than two marks on the back of your right hand, and never make the second mark until you have eight marks on your left! The marks will wash off at the end of each day, and you can begin a new record in the morning. You will be able to keep a permanent record of how well you are doing, and how well it relates to your weight loss, on your daily 28-Day Metabolic Breakthrough record forms (pp. 105–35).

Using the AC List

The AC list is loaded with complex-carbohydrate, high-fiber foods—whole grains, fruits, vegetables, and legumes. You can easily translate your choices from this list into the Four Food Group Plan recommended by leading nutritionists. Four servings of grains, cereal foods, or legumes plus two vegetables and two fruits will do it. But you really don't need to limit yourself in this way. Eight servings are actually your *minimum*—the more you learn to substitute fruits, vegetables, and grains for those densely caloric DC foods, the better.

The best way to assure that you are getting sound nutrition is to choose a wide variety of foods from the AC list. How about some grain foods for breakfast, two vegetables for dinner, and fruit with lunch, after dinner, and for snacks? *Always carry fruit wherever you go to make an AC/DC substitution.*

When you add about 6 ounces of lean meat, fish, or fowl (or use some of my complementary protein dishes, which combine legumes with grains or small amounts of meat or cheese), and when you add a couple of servings of foods high in calcium (e.g., milk products other than butter), you will assure yourself of obtaining adequate amounts of all the essential nutrients.

THE AC LIST

GRAINS, LEGUMES, AND TUBERS

all whole grains—wheat, rye, corn, barley, rice, and oats—as bread, cereals, and pasta
hominy
lentils

beans and peas, dried and cooked (black-eyed peas; kidney, lima, navy beans; baked beans; split peas)
potatoes, white or sweet
yams

VEGETABLES

asparagus
bean sprouts
beans, green or wax
broccoli
cabbage
cauliflower
celery
chickory
lettuce
mushrooms
okra
parsley
pepper, green and red
pimiento
artichoke
beets

carrots
peas, green
cucumber
eggplant
endive
escarole
greens of all kinds (beet, chard, collard, kale, mustard, spinach, turnip)
radish
romaine
sauerkraut
summer squash
tomato
zucchini
pumpkin

| rutabaga | turnip |
| winter squash | |

FRUITS

apples	figs	all berries
oranges	bananas	raisins
melon	mango	grapes
grapefruit	pears	cherries
dates	pineapple	apricots
dried prunes	peaches	papaya

Using the DC List

DC foods are dense in calories, which means that they have many calories relative to their other nutritional content of vitamins, minerals, and fiber. They are high in fat, and are usually processed. That is, their grains have been deprived of fiber, and often sugar is a major ingredient. Nutritionists sometimes refer to the calories in DC foods as "empty calories."

Alcohol, which has 7 calories per gram, and no other nutritional value, is included in the DC category. So are all soft drinks, since they are "straight" sugar.

As you will note from the list, DC foods are counted in terms of allowances rather than servings. While the total calories in each allowance may vary because these foods contain other ingredients, the number of calories from fat, sugar, or alcohol in each allowance is in the vicinity of 100.

You won't go wrong with two allowances from the categories listed below. Make sure you reach eight servings from the AC list before you add the second from the DC list, however.

It's best to consider those three teaspoons of fat or oil for spread, cooking, or flavoring as the number one choice in your daily DC allowance. Add the second allowance—one of those desserts, for example—only after you have had eight servings of AC foods.

Although it is usually not necessary to eliminate all of these snack and dessert foods to achieve a 1- to 3-pound weekly weight loss when you implement the other steps in the 28-Day Metabolic Breakthrough Plan, women who find it difficult to lose weight and who want the safest and quickest loss can eliminate that second DC food on a temporary basis. It (and more) will fit nicely back into your maintenance plan after you reach your desired weight.

THE DC LIST

alcohol (4 oz. wine, or the equivalent)

candy (reg.-size bar)

snack foods (potato chips, Fritos, granola bars— small-size package)

soft drinks (8 oz.)

desserts (serving of cake, pie, two cookies)

butter, margarine, oil (one allowance equals 3 t. daily)

ice cream (½ cup)

7

PHYSICAL ACTIVITY: A LITTLE GOES A LONG WAY

Six years ago, Phyllis was thirty-nine years old and, at 5 feet 8½ inches tall, weighed 192 pounds. Her eating diaries when she began her program indicated that she was consuming around 1950 calories per day.

Today, at forty-five years of age, she weighs 147 pounds and still eats approximately 1950 calories each day.

How come?

Each day Phyllis does something which, on the average, burns off the same number of calories her body used to require just to keep that 45 pounds of fat in her fat cells alive.

End result: she is 45 pounds lighter but still eats just as much as she did six years ago.

Phyllis has discovered something about physical activity that is not appreciated by many health professionals or overweight persons. You see, it is not how much activity is necessary to lose *X* number of pounds that is important. *It's what you have to do each day to keep all that excess weight off, once you lose it, that counts.* Without realizing it, you, too, just like Phyllis, are just *minutes* a day away from staying slim and fit for life.

Of course, the value of physical activity is great while you are losing weight as well. When you are in the process of losing weight, physical activity stimulates your metabolism, compensates for any metabolic conservation brought on if you do restrict your food intake, and helps prevent those plateaus and those annoying problems caused by water retention. You can say goodbye to those irritable moods and the discouragement you usually experience when you are several weeks into your ordinary weight-loss diets.

But the real value—the ultimate goal—of the Metabolic Breakthrough Plan is to show you how you can eat just as much as you do today and not regain a single pound once you reach your weight goal.

Your situation as of today is illustrated on the left side of Figure 7-1. As an overweight person—say, 25 to 50 pounds overweight—only about 100 to 200 calories of your total daily intake of food is going toward keeping your fat cells alive. Fat cells are not particularly active in a metabolic sense; they don't require anywhere near

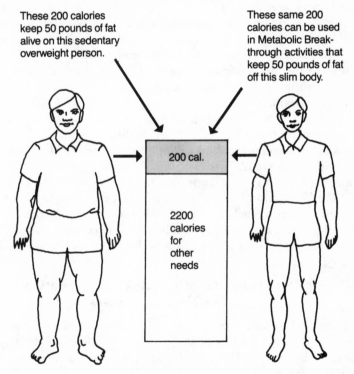

These 200 calories keep 50 pounds of fat alive on this sedentary overweight person.

These same 200 calories can be used in Metabolic Breakthrough activities that keep 50 pounds of fat off this slim body.

200 cal.

2200 calories for other needs

FIGURE 7-1. The overweight person is using 200 calories of the day's total intake of 2400 to support 50 extra pounds of fat. The slender person is using the same 200 calories each day in Metabolic Breakthrough physical activity. His total intake is the same, but he stays 50 pounds lighter than the fat person.

the calories just to stay alive that your heart, liver, kidneys, muscles, and nerve cells require. If you are a woman eating around 1800 calories each day, or a man at 2400, perhaps just 10 percent of your daily intake, that small fraction represented by the shaded portion of the bar between the figures, is actually being used to maintain as much as 50 pounds of excess weight.

When you reach the end of the 28-Day Metabolic Breakthrough Plan, your new situation is represented by that slimmer body at the right in Figure 7-1. When you reach your goal weight, you will have reprogrammed your body to burn the same number of calories, on the average, that it now takes to maintain your fat cells. The end result is *permanent weight control.*

Of course, it is not necessary (nor is it even possible) to figure out the *precise* number of calories you are using to support your excess fat. You simply start making the eating and activity changes required by the Metabolic Breakthrough Plan and arrive at your new balance through practical experience.

If you haven't reached your goal weight in 28 days—and it may take five or six months if you have 50 pounds to lose—you will nevertheless be firmly entrenched in the life-style that will get you there and keep you there. You will find that losing weight at the rate I recommend, that is, 8 to 10 pounds or so per month, makes permanent weight management much easier than weight management after a low-calorie, quick-loss diet. Just continue to follow the program until you reach your goal, using the dietary recommendations I have already made and any of the maximum metabolism improvement activities that I describe in Chapters 8 through 10.

Going From Fat to Thin: The Inside Information on Your Metabolic Processes

Compared with thinner, active people, fat, sedentary people are as different on the insides of their bodies, in their metabolic processes, as they are on the outside, in their more easily observable physical characteristics.

As you follow the 28-Day Metabolic Breakthrough Plan, you are going to start changing from a "fat" to a "thin" metabolism, as well as in diameter and circumference.

Take a look at Figure 7-2. In the "fat" metabolism depicted on

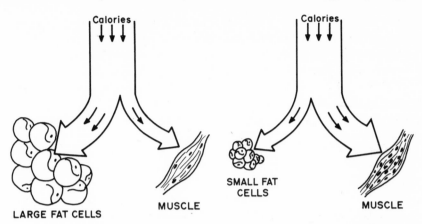

FIGURE 7-2.   Distribution of daily energy input between fat cells and muscle systems. The "fat" metabolism pictured on the left shunts a larger percentage of calories into its fat cells, compared with the active "thin" metabolism on the right. See the text for a full explanation.

the left, a large proportion of the calories from food get shunted off to your fat cells after every meal. That's because you never elevate that "fat" metabolism above the sitting or *resting level,* as it is more technically called. You never use up the glycogen that your body stores in your muscles and liver, which your body must use for fuel in much greater amounts every time you move around than it uses when you sit still.

For example, while you are sitting still, reading this book, a woman will be using about 60 to 70 calories per hour, a man around 80 or 90. That's about all you need while you are performing any sedentary work. This means that every time you eat, especially after that LARGE meal, your system has been forced to set up mechanisms (develop the hormones and enzymes) to get calories into your fat cells—and, by the way, to keep plenty of excess calories in storage.

The "thin" metabolism on the right uses energy quite differently. Each day, several hundred calories are used in physical activity. Part of the fuel you use for that activity, the glycogen part, is stored in your liver and muscle cells. So, they get depleted of their essential fuel each time you move. The key to developing a "thin" metabolism lies in the fact that *the priority for energy from your food is in your muscles and liver when they have been depleted by activity.* Thus, after meals, the active muscles and liver grab and store a larger part of your calories and these calories never see the insides of your fat cells at all.

Every single day, as you progress through the Metabolic Breakthrough Plan, going from fat to thin, your system is going to be making many changes[1]:

1. Your muscles will be manufacturing more and larger energy-producing sites. These mitochondria, as they are called, can be seen under the microscope and such changes have been verified in the laboratory. Your muscles will also begin to store more energy in the form of glycogen. Active muscles can as much as double their energy-storage capacity.

2. The myoglobin content of your muscles will increase. Myoglobin in the muscle, like hemoglobin in the bloodstream, combines with oxygen. Since you will be burning more fuel in your muscles, your system will adapt to give you a better supply of oxygen inside each of your active muscles so you can burn that fuel more easily.

3. Hormones and enzymes involved in energy utilization will increase. During and after activity, the secretion of fat-mobilizing hormones—for example, the catecholamines—will go up. Your fat cells will lose more and more of their fat content, while your active muscle cells, which use a mixture of fat and glucose (converted from glycogen) for fuel, get more proficient at grabbing that fat and burning it up.[2]

4. As your fat cells get smaller and the muscle cells more active, hormone and enzymatic activities involved in fat storage decrease. One of the most important health benefits of this change is an increase in your body cells' sensitivity to the action of insulin. As a person gains weight and fat cells get larger and larger, they become resistant to the action of insulin, which is one of the hormones that enables the transport of energy from the bloodstream into your body cells. This resistance leads to a condition known as hyperinsulinism, or an elevation in insulin level. This condition is often a precursor to adult onset diabetes.

When you become active and eat according to the principles I have already presented in this book, your system will no longer have to struggle to get those excess calories into your fat cells. So, insulin levels fall.[3,4]

Perhaps 80 percent of adult onset diabetes can be controlled or prevented with proper diet and exercise. *

In summary, the goal of the 28-Day Metabolic Breakthrough Plan is to change your body from a warehouse for fat to a veritable furnace for burning calories. And the key to permanent weight control lies in your ability to begin burning the same number of calories each day, on the average, that you now use to keep your fat cells full of fat.

*The 28-Day Metabolic Breakthrough Plan is as beneficial for the treatment of adult onset diabetes as it is for simple obesity, but you must consult with your physician in order to integrate it with your present treatment if you suffer from diabetes. Any unsupervised change in medication, diet, or activity levels in this condition, or in any other medical condition, can be dangerous.

8

THE METABOLIC
BREAKTHROUGH ACTIVITIES

"Which activities are best for weight control?"

"When is the best time for exercise?"

"How much do I have to do?"

These are the questions I am asked most frequently by people who want to maximize the calorie-burning value of every minute they spend in physical activity. Often these questions come from people who have become disenchanted with the value of exercise in weight control and have dropped out of exercise classes because the payoff didn't seem to be worth the effort. When I inquire about the details of their programs, I can understand and sympathize with them—their programs really weren't worth their efforts.

And that's because, when it comes to weight control, a maximum metabolic benefit approach to physical activity can be quite different from the approach that many fitness leaders take in their aerobic dance or calisthenics classes. Many leaders will work you to the limit of your endurance in short bursts of activity, but spend a major part of your time warming up for the workout, and relaxing at the end. A maximum benefit approach is also quite different from the one a coach might take in building a high level of athletic skill, strength, or endurance.

In these next three chapters I am going to discuss the general principles that underlie the best answers to "which," "when," and "how much" physical activity it takes for maximum metabolic improvement. Specific programs follow, but I think it is very important that you understand the principles first so that you can be as flexible as you like in developing any program of physical activity that will suit your unique interests, talents, and temperament.

Which Activities Are Best?

Here is the most important guideline and the fundamental principle of the 28-Day Metabolic Breakthrough Plan: *continuous WHOLE-BODY MOVEMENT burns the most calories with the least amount of perceived effort.*

When you use the large muscles in your legs and buttocks to propel your body through space, that's when you get the biggest payoff for your time and effort.

Unfortunately, many fitness leaders do not fully realize the importance of this principle. They may spend far too much of a person's limited time in toning, strengthening, or stretching exercises. Other, "celebrity-style" weight-control experts have you rotating your hips or swinging your arms until you think they're about to fall off, or grinding your bottom against the floor doing "tootsie-rolls." Of course, these exercises have some conditioning value and many persons find the TV shows entertaining, but when it comes to burning calories you're squandering your time. *You will burn 50 to 100 percent more calories just taking a walk than you will burn doing any of the exercises I have just mentioned.*

How can a simple physical activity like walking feel so much easier than exercises of the calisthenic variety and yet burn so many more calories?

When you do arm swings you move perhaps 10 to 20 percent of your body weight. It feels hard because you are using the relatively small muscles of your upper body in unaccustomed work. You tire in just a few minutes, and while these exercises help tone your upper body, you accomplish relatively little in terms of burning calories.

In contrast, with every walking step you take, you move your *entire* body weight—that's many more times the weight of your arms. It feels easier because you are using the largest and strongest muscles of your body. You are much more accustomed to this walking movement and, once in motion, your forward momentum helps you along. Furthermore, the biomechanical working relationship of your walking muscles to your body is better than that of the arms for arm swings, so you end up moving much more weight and obtaining twice the caloric benefit, with a fraction of the perceived effort.

There are other metabolic benefits that come from whole-body movement in addition to the ease with which you burn calories during physical activity itself.

After you have moved for a certain period of time, at a certain minimal intensity, your body keeps right on working for several hours afterward in order to repair and regenerate tissue in the muscles you have used, to get rid of the waste products generated by your exercise, and to restore the resting energy supply of glucose and fat in your tissues. In the 28-Day Metabolic Breakthrough Activity Program I will show you how to obtain easily an elevation in your metabolic rate that may last from two to six hours after you have finished being active. You may burn 20 percent more calories just sitting still for the subsequent two hours, and perhaps 10 percent more for the next two to four hours, than you would have burned without having been active.

The post-exercise calorie-burning effects of vigorous physical exercise can be rather dramatic. After an intense workout, athletes may sustain a 25 percent increase in resting metabolism for a full twenty-four hours. It may remain 10 percent higher for an additional twenty-four hours, even without further exercise.[1] And perhaps the lack of this effect is one of the reasons so many athletes begin to gain weight when they cease practicing and performing at such high intensities.

You and I, of course, are not aiming for such extreme effects. Later on, when I answer the question "How much?", I will explain the time and intensity factors through which you can obtain prolonged metabolic elevation in an enjoyable way, and with enough payoff to ensure that you will continue being active for the rest of your life.

For now, it is important to emphasize that most overweight persons cannot achieve this benefit from any activity outside of continuous whole-body movement, and it cannot be obtained from activity plans that do not meet the minimum requirements that I am going to spell out for you.

A 28-Day Metabolic Breakthrough Program can be constructed using any one or more of a variety of activities. At the start of your program, however, the two best whole-body activities are

1. walking and
2. rebounding on a minitrampoline.

After walking and bouncing, the next-best activities are

3. swimming and
4. bicycling.

Almost everyone in reasonable health can move right out in any one of these top four activities and begin to reap the best in the way of metabolic benefits with little, if any, risk of injury.

You may wonder why I have listed these activities in this particular order. It's quite simple. Walking is the most convenient activity and easily ranks highest at the start of the program because the number of calories you burn is greatest in terms of the effort you put into it. Brisk walking for a previously sedentary person is both the safest and the quickest way to alter a "fat" metabolism.

Rebounding is second because it is just as easy, although not quite as interesting and enjoyable as taking pleasant walks around your neighborhood or countryside. The main reason I always recommend that people in our program consider owning a rebounder is that, once you have one, there is *never* any excuse for not burning those calories that will keep you slim and fit. No matter what the weather or time of day, you have the rebounder in the corner of your bedroom or in front of the TV. Furthermore, almost everyone prefers the rebounder to a stationary bicycle; you can do many more interesting things with it, as you will discover in Chapter 16, where I describe a specific program of rebounding that is safe for everyone and that will burn just as many calories as walking or even running.

Swimming comes third because, while it may be about the best overall exercise in terms of working your entire body and because of its lack of stress on your weight-bearing joints, it is quite inconvenient for most people. And few people become expert enough to swim continuously for long enough to obtain maximum metabolic improvement benefits. Furthermore, I have long suspected that swimming tends to conserve a layer of surface body fat in order to protect you from the temperature difference between your body and the water. In any event, research shows that even competitive swimmers do maintain more body fat than other competitive athletes.[2]

Bicycling ranks fourth because it, too, like swimming, is rather inconvenient in most locales. There are traffic and the weather to be considered in cities. In addition, most people do not feel safe riding at speeds that will give metabolic benefits equivalent to walking. Even if they could, it is hard to maintain the same steady pace that you can with walking or bouncing. And finally, indoor, stationary bicycling often proves to be boring and rather uncomfortable. If you do wish to give stationary bicycling a try, or if you already own one that's been gathering dust in the corner because it hurts your bottom to use it for any length of time, I suggest you purchase what is called a "tractor" seat. This very comfortable seat may make all the difference in the world in your willingness to use your stationary bicycle if the seat that came with it is too tiny, narrow, and hard as a rock.

You are, of course, not limited to these four top-rated activities. You can apply maximum benefit principles to aerobic dancing of all varieties and the racquet sports. You simply have to find the right dance class or dance at home, or become moderately proficient in one of the racquet sports. All of these activities will work if you spend most of your time moving around briskly and not standing still.

Later on, as you lose weight and increase your fitness, you may want to consider an occasional jog as part of your routine, since this is the most convenient and efficient activity for burning calories and obtaining long-lasting metabolic benefits. It is not recommended at the start of the 28-Day Metabolic Breakthrough Plan for anyone more than 10 or 15 pounds overweight because of the risk of injury to the weight-bearing joints.

In summary, the best activities for making a metabolic breakthrough involve continuous whole-body movement. Walking or bouncing on a minitrampoline is the best way to start. You can end up with any activity you like, however, if you follow the principles I outline in the next two chapters.

9

THE AFTERNOON HIGH, OR THE TIME-OF-DAY FACTOR AND YOUR METABOLISM

"When is the best time for activity?"

The best answer to "when" is always "anytime—anytime that's convenient and that feels good."

But, if you are the kind of person who doesn't lose weight easily, or if you want to speed your loss, then certain times of the day can be better than others.

Research with both animals and humans indicates that you tend to burn the greatest number of calories in any given activity when your metabolic rate is already at a high point.

Human beings have two naturally occurring high points in their metabolic rates each day: late afternoons and after meals. If you get active at these naturally occurring high points, you may burn 10 percent or more calories than you would with the same activity at some other time.

The Afternoon High

Each day, your metabolic rate varies in cyclic fashion—it falls to its lowest point early in the morning, begins to rise when you awaken, continues to rise throughout the day, and begins to fall sometime after dinner. Most people reach their high points between 4:00 and 8:00 P.M.

Research with animals suggests that, when your metabolism is already naturally elevated, the "ceiling" seems to open up, so that it may go even higher in response to the same intensity of movement than it might earlier in the day.[1] When it comes to people, one recent study actually suggests that this effect may be greater for those who are overweight than for people of average weight.[2] This 10 percent boost can burn off the energy equivalent of several pounds of fat each year.

If you are one of those persons who has a gargantuan evening appetite, late afternoon activity may have yet another benefit. *It acts as a temporary appetite suppressant.* Therefore, if you tend to chomp away at night, for social reasons or just to reduce the tensions of the day, activity before dinner can help regulate your appetite so that you will be less likely to overeat at this time.

It works in the following ways: When you take a brisk walk (or jump about on that minitrampoline with the program I will outline for you) stored fat pours out of your fat cells and begins to circulate in your bloodstream on its way to supply your muscles with the necessary fat portion of their fuel mixture. Similarly, stored sugar flows out of your liver since your muscles need a mixture of both sugar and fat to do their work.

This elevation of both sugar and fat in your bloodstream mimics the blood content after meals, when the fat and sugar from your food are being circulated. The increase in fat and sugar content is sensed by the appetite centers in your brain, which then turn off their hunger signals.

Thus, physical activity in the late afternoon for persons who overeat from 4:00 P.M. to midnight can act as a double-edged sword in the battle for weight control: you are using your own stored sugar and fat supplies to *turn off your hunger signals as you go about losing weight,* rather than using the fat and sugar in the food you might otherwise have eaten to satisfy your hunger, and which would at the very least have kept you fat if it did not contribute to a further weight gain.

As you increase in fitness and increase the intensity and duration of physical activity, even greater temporary appetite-suppressing effects can be obtained from three other possible sources:

1. As your stored body fat is being metabolized for energy, certain by-products called ketones are being formed. In some people these ketones have an additional appetite-suppressing effect

that can last for several hours. You can create a considerable quantity of ketones with a thirty- to forty-five-minute walk before dinner.[3]

2. The hormones, such as catecholamines, that mobilize your body fat for fuel, may also play a role in turning off hunger signals.

3. The elevation in body temperature that accompanies activity at Metabolic Breakthrough Intensity, which I discuss in Chapter 11, is also considered to depress appetite.[4]

But now I know you may be worried if you cannot normally be active in the late afternoon or evening. You needn't be. If you happen to be what is called a "morning person," and if that is the only time you can fit some activity into a busy schedule, research has shown that your metabolism is already more elevated compared with the "evening person." Therefore, if you wake up raring to go in the morning, your body is signaling a higher than average metabolic rate. So, get up and go! You are already much higher in comparison with your total daily range, and it's much better to get moving than not to move at all. As I will explain more fully in Chapter 11, where I discuss the Metabolic Breakthrough Intensity Principle, body movement *at any time* can leave a residual metabolic elevation for several hours.

The After-Meal High

The second point at which your metabolism is naturally elevated really occurs several times a day—after meals.

Each time you eat, your body revs up in the process of digestion (this is the "thermic effect of food" that I spoke of earlier). Some studies show that if you take a walk after meals, you can increase this heat-generating effect, especially after large meals. If the process of digestion normally uses up about 10 to 15 percent of the caloric value of your meal, a fifteen-minute walk after that meal can push this cost up by another 10 percent. In effect, that walk can double the calories used in the digestive process.[5]

Consider a 1000-calorie meal: a walk after such a meal each day can push up the caloric cost in terms of the thermic effect as much as 100 calories. That alone is worth 10 pounds of fat a year.

Although some studies show that walking after meals may not increase the thermic effect for all obese people,[6] *it seems to have some special therapeutic value for persons with the greatest difficulty losing weight.*

If you believe that you can't lose weight on anything but a starvation diet, or if you have already used such diets in the past, either you may have been born with a slow metabolism or, after using a low-calorie diet, your body may have reduced its metabolic needs. At the start of your personal Metabolic Breakthrough Program, *walking after meals may be the very best means of turning your system around.*

Walking after meals has some special, quick-acting metabolic effects. I have observed this clinically in persons who cannot lose weight efficiently on 1000 calories, or even less. In addition to capitalizing on the thermic effect, that after-meal walk may change some fundamental process involved in fat storage. Activity after meals reduces the number of calories that your body needs to transport into your fat cells following eating. When you go for a walk after eating, you mobilize fat-burning hormones and enzymes and your muscles start gobbling up some of the calories you have just consumed. This may, in turn, decrease the body's need for large amounts of fat-storing hormones and enzymes. I can only speculate on the mechanism, but, whatever it is, walking after meals works to speed weight loss when all else short of semi-starvation fails.

I recommend walking at a moderate pace after meals because it is the easiest and most convenient thing to do for people with a stubborn weight problem, but any activity equivalent in intensity can be used, such as gentle rebounding. Whatever you choose, just keep the felt intensity of the activity equivalent to your feeling while walking at a moderate pace.

In summary, if you have a stubborn weight problem, or want to turn your system around after the metabolic slowdown brought on by low-calorie dieting, capitalize on your natural metabolic highs: activity in the late afternoon and walking at a moderate pace after meals are two of the best ways to do this.

10

HOW MUCH ACTIVITY IS ENOUGH?

At the end of your 28-Day Metabolic Breakthrough Plan you will be burning the same number of calories it now takes to support your excess fat.

When it comes to weight control, that is the very best answer there is to the question, "How much activity is enough?"

But, what does that answer really mean in practice?

Let me give you an example, and then I'll show you how to figure it out for yourself.

When Carol entered the Vanderbilt Weight Management Program, weighing 180 pounds, her eating diaries showed that she was eating approximately 2000 calories per day. Today she weighs 135 pounds and still eats approximately 2000 calories.

Each day, in her physical activity program, she burns the same number of calories it used to take to keep 45 pounds of unwanted excess fat alive, before she began her Breakthrough program.

The result is that she can eat just as she did before and not regain any weight.

In other words, when you burn at least as many calories as it now takes to keep your oversized fat cells alive, you can have perfect assurance that you will never regain any of the weight you lose in your Breakthrough program.

Without consciously realizing it or planning it that way, this was the principle I discovered over twenty years ago, after a minor coronary, when my physician said to me, "Lose weight and get active." I took up tennis. Within a month I was playing every day and burning up at least as many calories as it was taking to keep my extra 75 pounds of fat alive. I would cut back on my food (to around 1800 calories) for three to four weeks at a time, losing between 10 and 15 pounds each time. *I never regained any weight after each period of caloric restraint, until, after about a year and a half, I reached my desired weight.* *

During the periods in between my temporary "diets," my physical activity burned up at least as many calories as it had previously taken to maintain any of the fat I had lost. Thus, I would not regain any weight.

I eat more today than I ever did as a fat man during the first thirty-five years of my life. I average an hour a day in some sort of physical activity and burn a good 500 calories more in that hour than it would take to keep my vital processes going if I just sat still. As you will see in a moment, this permits me to eat much more per day than the average sedentary male.

But the real question at this point is, "What will it take for you?"

To answer that question, I will assume that you don't want to eat more than you do right now. You just want to weigh 20, 30, maybe even 50 or 75 pounds less, and come out even.

It takes perhaps 100 calories a day to support 20 or 25 pounds of fat on the human body. Thus, if you are up to 20 or 25 pounds overweight, you probably need to burn about 100 extra calories a day in physical activity to keep that much weight off after you lose it. Your total caloric intake could remain pretty much the same as it is today.

If you are up to 40 or 50 pounds overweight you will need to burn about 200 extra calories a day, and if you are 65 to 75 pounds overweight, I estimate that it will take about 300 calories a day to stay even with your present intake and keep your weight off.

Of course, when you combine my dietary recommendations with the Metabolic Breakthrough Activity Program, you will also be gaining metabolic benefits from changes in your eating habits. When you adhere to the AC/DC ratio each day, and have two servings of fiber foods with each meal, you may prevent about 100 calories from ever reaching your fat cells. Once you reach your weight goal, with full implementation of the program, you may find yourself *exceeding* your present consumption by several hundred calories, just as I do.

*See Appendix A, "How Much Should You Weigh?", for a discussion on the topic of desirable weight.

This is no idle statement fabricated out of "thin" air. A recent study at Stanford University showed that active persons between the ages of 35 and 59 eat more by 500 to 600 calories a day and weigh about 25 to 30 pounds less than sedentary persons.[1] The active subjects in the study actually reported eating 40 to 60 percent more calories per pound of body weight than the fatter, inactive persons.

This study is of special interest to me as a former fat person. The active subjects belonged to an informal running group and I suspect that not too many of them had ever been as fat as I. Perhaps they were naturally thin persons whose caloric intake would have been higher even if they were not running five to seven days a week and averaging between thirty-five and forty miles in that period. One might still ask, "Can a really fat person ever look forward to eating as much as those skinnies and not regain his weight?"

So, I compared my own mileage per week, and my weight, height, and caloric intake from eating records that I have kept periodically, with the averages reported in that study for persons who for the most part had probably never had a serious weight problem.

This is what I found: The average male in the study, although about 10 years younger than I, was within half an inch of my height and 4 pounds of my weight (5 feet 10½ inches, 154 pounds).

And this next figure I could hardly believe—the average reported caloric intake of the males in the study, taken from food records and an interview with a dietitian, was 2959 calories per day. My own records, taken over a two-week, weight-stable period in which I weighed and measured every mouthful of food, show 2960 calories per day.

What about the sedentary males in the study? In line with national averages, they were found to be consuming 2361 calories per day, at a body weight of around 180 pounds.

Thus, just like those runners, I am eating 600 calories a day *more* than the average sedentary man. And that average sedentary male, eating 600 calories less than I do, weighs a good 25 pounds more than I do. While I cannot verify this statement because I did not keep eating records twenty years ago, I feel sure that I am eating several hundred calories more each day at the present time than I did when I weighed 230 pounds.

The story is exactly the same for the women in the study. The active women were averaging 2386 calories per day, and, at just over

120 pounds, weighed about 30 pounds *less* than the inactive women who were eating only 1871 calories per day.

How about that? Wouldn't you like to eat 500 calories more per day and weigh 30 pounds less?

You may, of course, be wondering why I present a study comparing runners with nonrunners when I have already issued a warning about running for overweight people. I present this study only for illustrative purposes—you can accomplish an identical result with any number of physical activities that meet the metabolism improvement guidelines that I am spelling out for you in this chapter.

Take a look at Table 10-1. It contains a list of various whole-body activities that you can use in your own 28-Day Metabolic Breakthrough Plan, with the calories burned in each 5 minutes of activity. Just add up 5-minute periods until you reach your total—it will take about 100 calories' worth of extra activity to keep off each 20 to 25 pounds of surplus weight that you are presently lugging around with you each day. Use any combination of activities that appeals to you.

While I want to encourage you to experiment with many of these activities and discover the ones that give you the greatest satisfaction, I find that most people prefer walking, at least to start, and even when they find some other activities that they include for variety, walking continues to play a major role in their activity programs.

You will see in Table 10-1 that each 5 minutes of walking at 3 MPH, which is a moderate pace, burns about 22 calories. When you up the pace to 4 MPH, which is considered "brisk," you burn around 33 calories every 5 minutes. (These are averages for a person weighing between 150 and 160 pounds—the heavier you are, the more you burn.)

The average woman will walk at 3 MPH when she takes 20 to 21 steps every 10 seconds. The average man takes only about 16 to 17 steps every 10 seconds to reach that pace because the male stride tends to be longer.

At 4 MPH the average woman takes about 27 to 28 steps every 10 seconds, while the man is up to 22 or 23.

It's very easy to arrive at a good approximation of your pace by simply counting your steps as you time yourself for 10 seconds. You will have it down pat in just one or two counts.

TABLE 10-1
Energy Expenditure in Physical Activities*

ACTIVITY	MINUTES OF ACTIVITY					
	5	10	15	30	45	60
Walking						
moderately, 3 miles per hour	22	44	66	132	198	264
briskly, 4 miles per hour	33	66	99	198	297	396
Rebounding**						
brisk walking tempo,						
little foot lift	22	44	66	132	198	264
jogging tempo,						
foot lift of 4–6 inches	33	66	99	198	297	396
running, high knee						
lifts, or kicks	68	136	204	408	612	816
Badminton	34	68	102	204	306	408
Cycling						
leisure, 5.5 miles per hour	22	44	66	132	198	264
leisure, 9.4 miles per hour	35	70	105	210	315	420
Chopping wood						
average tempo	30	60	90	180	270	360
Dancing						
moderate tempo	18	36	54	108	162	216
continuous, intense aerobic	59	118	177	354	531	708
Gymnastics	23	46	69	138	217	276
Horseback riding						
trot, English style	39	78	117	234	351	468
Martial arts, judo, karate						
continuous drill	68	136	204	408	612	816
Rowing						
moderate pace	26	52	78	156	234	312
Running (flat surface)						
a mile in 11½ minutes	47	94	141	282	423	564
a mile in 9 minutes	68	136	204	408	612	816
a mile in 8 minutes	73	146	219	436	655	874
a mile in 7 minutes	81	162	243	486	729	972
a mile in 6 minutes	88	176	264	528	792	1056
a mile in 5½ minutes	101	202	303	606	909	1212
Skiing						
moderate, downhill	42	84	126	252	378	504
cross country	50	100	150	300	450	600

(continued)

TABLE 10-1 *(Continued)*

ACTIVITY	MINUTES OF ACTIVITY					
	5	10	15	30	45	60
Squash	74	148	222	444	666	888
Stair climbing						
down, rate of 1 step per second	17	34	51	102	153	204
up, rate of 1 step per second	72	144	216	432	648	864
Swimming						
continuous freestyle, slow	45	90	135	270	405	540
continuous freestyle, fast	55	110	165	330	495	660
Table tennis	24	48	72	144	216	288
Tennis						
singles	38	76	114	228	342	456

*Estimates taken from Martin Katahn, *The 200 Calorie Solution*, Norton, 1982. All values are approximate for a person weighing 154 pounds.
**Rebounding exercise must move at a faster pace than walking on a level surface because of the assist given to your movement by the springing action of the minitrampoline.

If you wish to be very exact, measure out a mile according to the odometer on your car, or go to a track. Three miles per hour is, of course, a mile in 20 minutes, and 4 miles per hour is a mile every 15 minutes. That breaks down to quarter-mile times of 5 minutes and 3 minutes and 45 seconds, respectively. You will be amazed at how quickly your body learns to "feel" these paces (or any others that you practice). Soon you will be able to walk within seconds of any speed you desire without ever consulting your watch. I think you will be rather impressed with your ability to match time with the rhythm of your movement.

When it comes to total time for activity, I always start out with participants in the Vanderbilt program by telling them to plan for a comfortable margin. After all, overweight people are periodically if not continually restraining their eating behavior in an effort to control their weight. It certainly would be nice to be done with that necessity once and for all, and to enjoy the good things in life without feeling worried or guilty. So, I think you, too, should plan from the onset of your program to develop the life-style that will erase forever most, if not all, of your need to worry about whether you are eating too much.

For this reason, the 28-Day Metabolic Breakthrough Plan builds everyone to a level of around 45 minutes of whole-body movement, on the average, each day. Our research shows that this will give most people up to about 50 pounds overweight a comfortable margin in their future caloric consumption.[2,3]

I emphasize 45 minutes of activity "on the average, each day" because you must orient yourself to a *daily* program, even though a day off each week is perfectly acceptable, and even desirable, if you have been particularly vigorous the day before or if you find yourself being active for longer than 45 minutes for several days. I usually take a day off from running or tennis each week, but I must admit that I find myself arranging to walk more on that day. I just don't feel as well, or work as well, if all I do is sit all day. Go by the way you feel, because a day off can be refreshing if you are tired from overexertion. Rest is especially important if you have a fever.

However, do not try to double up on activity—say, exercise 2 hours, three times a week—in order to come up with a satisfactory weekly average. You are truly in danger of hurting yourself physically under these conditions. Most accidents, muscle strains, and joint injuries occur when a person is tired. When it comes to weight control, a moderate amount almost every day, at an intensity that leaves you refreshed rather than exhausted, is the very best way.

11

THE INTENSITY PRINCIPLE

You must be active at a certain minimum intensity for a certain amount of time if you wish to obtain a prolonged elevation in your metabolic rate that keeps on burning fat long after you finish being active.

You must move about in any whole-body activity that requires your heart to beat between 70 and 90 percent of its maximum obtainable rate for at least thirty minutes.

Sounds complex, but it isn't.

All it takes for most overweight persons at the start of their 28-Day Metabolic Breakthrough Activity Program is a brisk walk, or the equivalent effort on a rebounder. You really don't need to worry about the technical details of your heart rate if you don't wish to. Just move along briskly at whatever level you can comfortably sustain for at least thirty minutes. You should be breathing harder, but not so hard that you couldn't continue a conversation if you wished to. Perspiration is an indication that you have raised your body temperature and metabolic rate. The intensity of movement should be high enough so that you finish pleasantly exhilarated, not exhausted.

How to Determine Your Metabolic Activity

I will, however, explain the technical procedure for evaluating your metabolic improvement activity. It is, in reality, quite simple. Do it just once or twice and it will provide lasting motivation to continue with your program. It will demonstrate to you that you are burning between 50 and 100 calories more during the next several hours after you finish your metabolic improvement activity each day than you would have otherwise.

There are several steps to the procedure:
1. Learning to take your pulse accurately.
2. Estimating your maximum obtainable heart rate.
3. Determining the 70 and 90 percent levels.
4. Monitoring your pulse at the appropriate times.

Step 1: Learning to Take Your Pulse

To take your pulse, place two fingers (not your thumb—it has a pulse of its own) over the radial artery or over the carotid artery. The radial artery lies on a line along the inside of your wrist leading toward your thumb. The carotid artery can be felt to the side of, and just behind, your Adam's apple.

Count the beats for ten seconds and multiply by 6. This will give you your heart rate in beats per minute.

For example, if you count 14 beats in ten seconds, 14 times 6 will give you a heart rate of 84 beats per minute.

Practice it a few times.

Step 2: Estimating Your Maximum Heart Rate

Theoretically, your maximum heart rate is obtained by subtracting your age from the figure 220. In reality, however, the fastest that your own heart might beat, under maximum effort in an all-out sprint for a couple of hundred yards, might be a little higher or lower than that figure. Since most of us are not in shape for such a test, we go by averages that have been obtained in experiments using large numbers of people of all ages.

It's obvious from the rule that our maximum heart rates decline with age; on the average, a person of thirty years of age will have a maximum obtainable rate of around 190 beats per minute, a person of fifty years of age will have a maximum rate of around 170, and little kids racing around the playground easily get their rates up over 200 or 210.

Calculate your own theoretical maximum heart rate by subtracting your age from 220.

For example, if your age is 43:

$$\begin{array}{r} 220 \\ -43 \\ \hline 177 \end{array}$$

This is your maximum obtainable heart rate.

To make it easy for you, a tabulation of maximum heart rates by age is presented in Table 11-1.

TABLE 11-1

Maximum Rates and Metabolism Improvement Ranges*

AGE	MAX. H.R. (BPM)	60% LEVEL (BPM)	70% LEVEL (BPM)	90% LEVEL (BPM)
20	200	120	140	180
25	195	117	137	176
30	190	114	133	171
35	185	111	130	167
40	180	108	126	162
45	175	105	123	158
50	170	102	119	153
55	165	99	116	149
60	160	96	112	144
65	155	93	108	140

*Taken from Martin Katahn, *The 200 Calorie Solution,* Norton, 1982, p. 89.

Step 3: Calculating Your 70- to 90-Percent Level

Multiply the figure you have obtained in Step 2 first by .70 and then by .90. This will give you your metabolism improvement range. Using the example in Step 2:

```
   177          177
 ×.70         ×.90
  124          159
```

The range in this example is from 124 to 159.

Again, to make it easy for you, these ranges by age are given in Table 11-1.

Step 4: Monitoring Your Pulse at the Appropriate Times

To demonstrate that you are obtaining maximum metabolic improvement through physical activity by prolonging an elevation in your metabolic rate, you use the following procedure:

1. Take your pulse before you begin your day's activity. This is your pre-exercise base rate. Make a record of it so that you will not forget it.

2. Take your pulse once in the middle of your activity session and once again at the end, to be sure that you have maintained an activity heart rate of at least 70 percent of maximum throughout.

3. Continue to record your pulse rate about once an hour for the next several hours thereafter.

If you have elevated your heart rate for at least thirty minutes to the 70 percent of maximum level or above, you will find that it stays somewhat elevated for two or more hours afterward—perhaps by 20 percent over your pre-exercise rate for an hour or two, and by 10 percent for some time after.

Although the correspondence between heart rate and metabolic rate is not perfect—that is, the percentage increase in heart rate may be somewhat more or less than the percentage increase in metabolic rate—any elevation following activity indicates an elevation in metabolism. As exercise increases in intensity and duration, the greater will be the post-activity elevation and the longer it will last. Following a thirty-minute walk at the 70 percent of maximum level, the minimum elevation that I have noted in women using walking as their metabolism improvement activity was approximately 10 percent two hours later.

Since I am able to run or jog faster and longer than persons entering our program, I have used myself as a subject in studies of heart rate after exercise. Following an hour's jog in which I do forty minutes at about 70 percent of my maximum heart rate, and twenty minutes between 80 and 90 percent of maximum, my heart rate remains elevated by 22 percent over my nonexercise resting baseline for about two hours (that may sound like a lot, but my resting pulse hovers between 42 and 48 beats per minute at five in the morning, and reaches 54 without exercise at five in the afternoon). Then, it gradually subsides over the next four hours to the level it would have been at if I hadn't exercised at all. I calculate that this elevation corresponds to about 100 extra calories over and above what I would have otherwise burned in that six-hour period of sitting still.*

*Heart rate over a wide range of exercise is a good indicator of our metabolic rate. However, the relationship of heart rate to metabolic rate is unique to each individual. It can be determined in the laboratory by measuring, simultaneously, the oxygen consumed and the associated heart rate as you perform a variety of different activities (e.g., walking, jogging, running at different speeds). Since 1 liter of oxygen is consumed during the burning of 4.82 calories, the amount of oxygen consumed tells us how many calories were burned in a given period of time. In some cases, the percentage change is quite close—a 10 percent increase in heart rate corresponds to a 10 percent increase in oxygen consumption. In other cases, especially in very fit individuals, a 10 percent increase in heart rate can reflect a 20 or 30 percent increase in oxygen consumption. This occurs because, with each beat, the heart of the fit person expels more blood, and the oxygen-carrying capacity of the blood as well as the utilization capacity of the muscle system are greater than those of the less fit person. (Continued on next page.)

Getting Started

During the first week of your 28-Day Metabolic Breakthrough Program it is important that you *start slowly*. Whatever activity you choose—walking, rebounding, swimming, or cycling—go at your most comfortable pace. If you take your pulse, you may find that it is only in the 60- to 70-percent range. That will be fine. There is no need to go higher at first—we use Week 1 to get in shape and to get over any little soreness that might occur if you have not been active for a long time. The 60-percent level, while not high enough to prolong an elevation in your metabolism for an extended period after activity, is still high enough to increase your cardiovascular endurance and to start building some muscular strength. It is safe even for persons in cardiac rehabilitation programs.

By the second week we get to the 70-percent level, and then we can build up to one daily period of thirty minutes in the 70 to 90 percent of maximum range. Persons using walking after meals will continue to make an exception to the intensity principle and walk at their most comfortable pace regardless of heart rate.*

We are now ready for explicit instructions for setting up your personal 28-Day Metabolic Breakthrough Nutrition Plan and Activity Program.

Except after vigorous activity, the heart rate at rest is not a very good indicator of metabolic rate. It is influenced by our moods, whether we have had an argument with someone, our stress levels, and by the things we have smoked or eaten, such as nicotine, alcohol, or caffeine. The same elevation of heart rate after an argument does not reflect nearly the same calorie consumption as if it had occurred during or after physical activity.

*While most healthy people certainly don't need their doctor's permission to go for a walk, if you have been leading a sedentary life, are more than 15 pounds overweight, and are over thirty-five years of age, or if you have any medical problem that has led to an adverse reaction to physical activity in the past, you should be sure to consult your physician and explain that you are going to build a program of *brisk* walking (or other activity of your choice).

If you develop anything more than slight soreness, or if any ache or pain from activity persists at the same or greater intensity for more than twenty-four hours, I also think you should get professional advice. Many slight problems caused by improper walking or jogging shoes, or other athletic equipment that doesn't quite suit you, can become major if not corrected early. Don't stint—buy the best equipment. And if you want an expert and honest fitness evaluation and personal supervision in your activity program, consult your local YMCA Fitness Director.

PART **II**

Breakthrough!

12

WHAT TO EXPECT FROM YOUR 28-DAY METABOLIC BREAKTHROUGH PLAN

When most persons think of losing weight, they have "going on a diet" uppermost in their minds. And, I suspect that you want to lose weight right now, too, or you would not be about to begin this program.

But the ultimate goal of the 28-Day Metabolic Breakthrough Plan goes way beyond weight loss. It's designed to bring about the changes in your life-style and in your body that will ensure permanent weight control without the need to keep on dieting.

I want to plant this goal firmly in your mind's eye:

By the fourth week of the 28-Day Metabolic Breakthrough Plan you will be burning enough calories to keep as much as 50 pounds of fat off your body forever.

Think about that for a moment. It is an entirely different mental orientation. It means that you, just like the formerly overweight persons from the Vanderbilt program who have lost 50 pounds or more, will soon be able to eat pretty much in accordance with your natural appetite and not regain weight.

So, set your sights on reaching your fat-burning goal first even if you have more pounds to take off than you can safely lose in one month. When you reach your fat-burning goal in the fourth week of the program, you can be confident that, as you continue to lose down to your desired weight, you will keep it off forever.

How fast will you lose? After a quick, initial loss that often approaches 3 to 5 pounds in the first week, women will settle down to an average loss thereafter that ranges between 1 and 3 pounds per week. The more overweight you are, the more you tend to lose. Men may lose twice as quickly as women because they have a larger fat-burning muscle mass than women to begin with, and their bodies are not gifted (or cursed) with the same ability to preserve surplus fat stores.

Weight loss starts quickly because, during the first few days, you can expect to lose a pound for every 500-calorie deficit between your energy intake and your energy expenditure.[1] This loss may consist of as much as 80 percent water, and it occurs as a result of a reduction in sodium intake and the burning of a relatively large proportion of stored glycogen in your body's fuel mixture. Then, gradually, as your body rids itself of all its excess water and you start burning a larger and larger percentage of fat, weight loss, as measured on your bathroom scale, appears to slow down.

This slowdown may have discouraged you in the past when you had simply gone on a diet and had nothing more than continued deprivation to look forward to. But there is no need for that now. As you proceed with the Metabolic Breakthrough Plan, you will be burning an increasing amount of fat and losing more and more weight out of your fat stores than ever before. This is illustrated in Figure 12-1. In Week 2 you lose more fat than in Week 1; in Week 3 you lose more fat than in Week 2; and in Week 4 you lose more fat than in Week 3. In Week 4 you reach your full fat-burning potential. Virtually all of the weight you lose thereafter is being permanently withdrawn from your fat cells.

In fact, our body composition studies at Vanderbilt show that people following the principles of the program actually lose *more* weight in fat than their scales can show. So will you. You will be adding to your fat-burning potential by increasing your lean muscle tissue by perhaps 1 pound with every 10 pounds of fat you lose.

Thus, when your scale shows 18 pounds lost, you may in reality have lost 20 pounds of fat.

Our findings are not at all unusual. I have examined the body composition changes and the components of weight loss in fifty-five different physical training studies to verify this point.* Our findings are seen in just about every study that comes close to following the principles of the 28-Day Metabolic Breakthrough Plan. They are

*I present the complete findings of this analysis in Chapter 21.

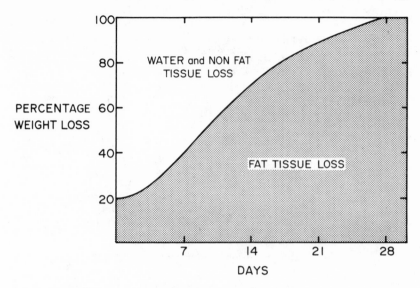

FIGURE 12-1. Approximate relative amount of water and lean tissue lost vs. fat lost as you progress through the 28-Day Metabolic Breakthrough Program. See the text for a full explanation.

illustrated in Figure 12-2. You can see that, by Week 4, and in the following weeks, your actual fat loss can be ever so slightly exceeding the amount of weight loss shown on your scale.

The end result is therefore very different from your low-calorie diets, which continue to force the body to use up part of its lean tissue for fuel. On low-calorie diets, especially those below 800 calories, as much as 35 to 45 percent of all the weight you lose may be important lean tissue. And that's terrible. It's self-defeating because, even at rest, your lean muscle tissue burns about three times the calories that fat tissue does. This means that low-calorie diets, by depleting your muscle mass, cause you to lose part of your fat-burning potential.

Of course, all of this just helps to explain the reason you may have found it so easy to gain weight after some of your previous diets.*

*Some popular commercial formula diets maintain that their powders contain just the right amount of nutrients to prevent the loss of lean tissue. In my opinion, from a careful study of the research literature, this is definitely not true. The literature shows that all persons will lose a considerable amount of lean tissue for about six

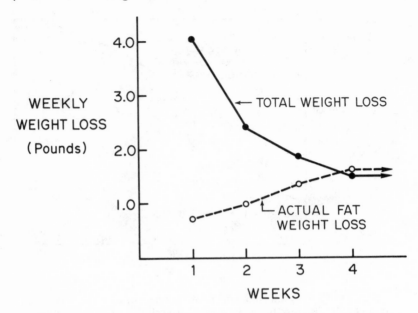

WEEKLY
WEIGHT LOSS
(Pounds)

FIGURE 12-2. A comparison of total weight loss and actual fat loss each week on the 28-Day Metabolic Breakthrough Plan. By Week 4, actual fat loss may exceed total weight loss. See the text for an explanation.

You can be confident that, when you lose weight following the Metabolic Breakthrough Activity Program on a daily basis and add-

weeks using any of these powdered diets. Then, on the *average*, they *may* come into "nitrogen balance." Since nitrogen is a component of protein, it is felt that when balance is achieved, and the body does not excrete more nitrogen than is contained in the formula, it is no longer losing muscle mass.

Much of the research quoted in the advertising used to support the claims of the popular formulas fails to mention the huge percentage of persons who never do achieve nitrogen balance—*it may reach 50 percent or even higher.* It means that a large number of people will be burning important tissue, not only from their skeletal muscle system, but from their hearts as well, as their bodies convert protein stores into glucose for fuel. Furthermore, the research quoted has on numerous occasions overlooked the fact that, after prolonged semi-starvation, the by-products of body-protein metabolism may be given off in the form of other compounds such as ammonia, not nitrogen. These other compounds can be more difficult to measure than nitrogen and they are given off in perspiration, which is not measured, as well as in the feces and urine. Unbiased investigators continually point out the dangers and self-defeating aspects of these diets.[2,3]

ing to your lean tissue mass, you can be increasing your overall energy needs each day.

Using Your Body Measurements

You will gain additional assurance that body composition changes are taking place, and that your fat-burning potential is increasing, by taking your body measurements each week and recording them on the forms provided.

Keeping body measurements can be a real morale booster because, at some point during weight loss, your body may attempt to conserve its weight by retaining water. It seems that fat cells are stubborn—they "don't like" to lose their mass, so they sometimes take in water to replace the fat you are burning.

You are still burning fat, but the water that is replacing it weighs more than the fat you are burning.

I am sure you've noticed this difference in weight between fat and water because fat floats on top of water and it rises to the top of your soups and stews. But you may not have made a connection to your own weight, which is this: because water is more dense than fat, the same weight in the water that may be temporarily replacing your fat is going to take up less space in your body cells. Your inches will continue to go down even though the scale doesn't. If you stick with the plan, your body finally realizes that you mean business and your fat cells release the water. Weight loss starts again with a bang —even if you haven't lost any weight for several days you will wake up one morning 2 or 3 pounds lighter.

Whenever you see a loss of inches over any period of time that shows little or no weight change, it means you are still losing fat and that you are continuing to build your fat-burning potential.

Be sure to keep a record of your body measurements each week in order to demonstrate these body composition changes in case you hit a plateau. Fortunately, such plateaus do not occur frequently on this program because both the Nutrition Plan and the Activity Program counter tendencies to retain water.

How to Deal with Cyclic Water Retention

Water retention attributable to the menstrual cycle can pose a problem for many women and lead to considerable puffiness. It is therefore important for women to realize that any associated weight gain is indeed due to water retention, but that fat burning—*real fat weight loss*—continues on the Metabolic Breakthrough Plan even though your scale weight may be increasing.

You can minimize water retention by avoiding salt and foods high in sodium (p. 149) and by maintaining your increased level of activity. Even under conditions of inactivity, your body loses almost as much water through the lungs during breathing and through perspiration as it does through the kidneys. By staying active you increase these channels of water loss significantly.

Continue to drink plenty of water (at least eight glasses per day) to stimulate the kidneys and elevate your metabolism. Also emphasize foods in your diet that have a natural diuretic action. These foods include fresh pineapple, melons, fresh asparagus and green vegetables, and citrus fruits, either peeled in sections or as juice. Both coffee and tea also have a slight diuretic action, but I recommend limiting your consumption of these beverages to about two cups a day to avoid irritating your stomach when you reduce your food intake.

You may have heard that vitamin B_6 also has some diuretic action. However, except for iron in the diets of women who tend to be low in this nutrient, I do not ordinarily recommend taking extra quantities of any single vitamin or mineral on a routine basis because vitamins and minerals work together. You can unbalance the natural ratio of nutrients that you obtain from an adequate diet when you drastically increase your intake of any single nutrient or special combination of nutrients beyond your body's natural needs. Other possible exceptions to this general rule apply to smokers, persons who consume large quantities of caffeine or alcohol, persons in situations of extremely high stress, women using birth control pills, or persons who cannot eat a mixed diet. A multiple vitamin and mineral capsule may be of value in such cases since the need for vitamin C and the B complex may be increased. Nevertheless, you should remember that vitamins and minerals in overdoses can have deleterious long-term effects on your metabolic processes. It is truly in your best interest not to take vitamin and mineral capsules that exceed the U.S. Recommended Dietary Allowances without guidance from a health professional trained in nutrition.

Special Help For Ex-smokers and Persons Who Plan to Quit

Smoking elevates your metabolism to the point where it burns an extra 100 to 200 calories a day. This, together with any other oral gratifications that smoking affords, means that it is very easy to gain weight when you quit. A gain of 12 to 20 pounds is not uncommon, and one woman who entered the Vanderbilt program had previously gained 37 pounds in one year after quitting.

When you stop smoking, your metabolic rate may fall between 5 and 10 percent. If you are a sedentary person and go on a low-calorie diet in order to control your weight when you quit smoking, *you lower your metabolic rate still further.* A conservative estimate would place the total loss in your daily metabolic needs at around 30 percent and it might be considerably more. Thus, you only increase your potential for gaining weight if you ever return to your customary level of food intake with this approach.

In contrast, if you have recently stopped smoking or plan to, the Metabolic Breakthrough Plan will not only completely compensate for any metabolic slowdown due to the lack of nicotine effects, it will have you burning several hundred calories more each day than you did as a smoker.

It is far healthier and far more effective to control your weight with the Breakthrough Plan than to continue smoking if you have been afraid to stop because of the potential for weight gain. If you desire to stop smoking, check with your physician, the American Heart Association, or the American Cancer Society for advice on how to successfully rid yourself of that habit.

13

HOW TO CHOOSE YOUR 28-DAY METABOLIC BREAKTHROUGH ACTIVITY PROGRAM

You begin with one of three programs designed to meet your personal needs.

The *Regular Program* is for men and women in good health who have not been active in the recent past. And it is safe even for persons who suffer from a variety of ills, including hypertension, diabetes, and mild arthritis, to mention a few, but if you suffer from any illness you should consult with your physician and obtain special instructions to adapt the program to your needs.*

The *Super Booster Program* is for persons who know from experience that they are slow losers. If you have had problems losing weight on sensible diets in the past, you may have been born with lower metabolic needs, or you may have lowered your needs through repeated dieting and a lack of activity. This can be remedied by starting with a schedule that will capitalize on natural highs in your daily metabolic rate and thereby maximize your weight loss. Within a few weeks you may find that your metabolic processes have speeded up to the point where special efforts are no longer neces-

---

*This program has been used safely and effectively with otherwise healthy individuals up to 125 pounds overweight. However, if you suffer from this degree of overweight I suggest that you consult with your physician before beginning any vigorous activity program, and that you proceed through the stages of the 28-Day Plan more slowly. Double the suggested lengths of time at each level—it is better to take eight weeks to reach the fat-burning goal of the Metabolic Breakthrough Plan than to hurt yourself along the way and never get there at all.

sary. Then you can become as flexible as you like with your schedule.

The *Advanced Program* is for persons less than 50 pounds overweight who have been involved in moderate activity programs once or twice a week, such as calisthenics or aerobic dance, a tennis game, or eighteen holes of nonmotorized golf. If this applies to you, you can begin immediately at a higher level.

Here is a summary of each program in some detail to provide you with an overview. Table 13-1, on page 85 at the end of this chapter, presents an outline for ready reference. Brief reviews are given with the record forms at the beginning of each week of the 28-Day Metabolic Breakthrough Nutrition Plan and Activity Program.

Regular Program

Week 1

Week 1 is a conditioning week. You will build up to 15 minutes of daily activity at whatever pace or intensity feels good to you and leaves you with no aches or pains. You can do it in

1. three 5 minute periods or
2. a 5- and a 10-minute period or
3. one 15-minute period each day.

Persons more than 50 pounds overweight, or anyone who has been very sedentary: aim for a total of 15 minutes at a *slow pace*. In walking, anything under 3 miles per hour (MPH) is considered a slow pace. From the psychological perspective, you are looking for comfort and minimal perceived effort. From a physical standpoint, because you are out of shape, or your degree of overweight might cause joint or muscular problems, you must go slowly enough to avoid injury.

Persons less than 50 pounds overweight, but generally sedentary: aim immediately for 15 minutes of activity at a *moderate pace*. In walking, a moderate pace is between 3 and 3.5 miles per hour, or from 17.5 to 20 minutes per mile. From a psychological standpoint, the effort "feels moderate," as though you could go all day as far as your breathing is concerned. Of course, in time, your legs would get tired and you would feel fatigued.

Week 2

In Week 2 you increase your pace to Metabolic Breakthrough Intensity. After a minute or two of moderate movement, you increase your pace gradually until you are moving at the maximum comfortable intensity that you could maintain for 15 minutes if you had to.

Persons less than 50 pounds overweight: your goal is 15 minutes of *brisk* activity.

Persons more than 50 pounds overweight: your goal is 15 minutes of *moderately paced* activity.

Brisk walking is from 3.5 to 4.5 miles per hour. Because of added weight, heavier persons will achieve heart rates at more moderate speeds that equal the heart rates of lighter persons moving at a brisk pace. So, the heavier you are, the sooner you will reach Metabolic Breakthrough Intensity. For people 50 pounds overweight, it tends to be at around 3 miles per hour.

Everyone can still break their activity up into convenient periods. You can use your bodily sensations or your heart rate to determine whether you are obtaining maximum metabolic benefits. Your breathing rate should increase, but not reach the point where you could not carry on a conversation if you wished to. If you finish exhausted rather than refreshed, you have overexerted. Your heart rate is your best guide: it should be at 70 percent of its maximum when you finish, and not higher than 90 percent (see pages 67–68). You should move about at a lower intensity for at least a couple of minutes when you finish, before you sit down. This will prevent blood from pooling in your legs and any feeling of lightheadedness.

Week 3

In Week 3 you increase activity to thirty minutes at Metabolic Breakthrough Intensity. If your schedule demands, it can be done in short periods, and you can take pleasure in knowing that you burn 20 to 25 calories with every five minutes of moderate activity and 30 to 35 calories with five minutes of brisk activity, compared with 5 to 7 in the sitting position. However, prolonged fat mobilization and continued elevation in your metabolic rate require about 30 minutes of continuous whole-body movement.

We are now working primarily for duration of activity—a full 30 minutes each day. Persons more than 50 pounds overweight may find it necessary to break up the activity more than will lighter persons. If you are more than 50 pounds overweight, take comfort in knowing that a *moderate* pace—just 3 miles per hour—is yielding the same metabolic improvement as the *brisk* pace for lighter persons. You are carrying more weight, which means that your workload equals that of persons who carry less but go faster. And don't worry, you'll catch up as your weight goes down.

Week 4

In Week 4 you increase to 45 minutes of daily activity at Metabolic Breakthrough Intensity. Heavier persons will find their cardiovascular and muscular endurance increasing dramatically and they will begin to pick up speed.

You can use any combination of time periods for activity—5, 10, 15, etc., minutes to reach the total of 45. Because prolonged calorie burning after activity requires about 30 minutes at Metabolic Breakthrough Intensity (a minimum of 70 percent of your maximum heart rate) I strongly recommend at least one period of 30 minutes of brisk activity each day, plus 15 more minutes obtained in any convenient way.

Whether or not you choose to do your activity all in one single session of 45 minutes, use as your guide to the appropriate pace the most vigorous intensity that you could muster and maintain for a full 45 minutes if you chose to; I want to emphasize that this means an intensity you could *maintain* for that period of time without ill effects. Most people start out too fast the moment anyone says "vigorous" in connection with activity. Modulate the intensity to the time, because the total time is the most important factor.

Forty-five minutes of activity will keep up to 50 pounds of fat from coming back into your fat cells after you reach desired weight. If you have more than 50 pounds to lose, but are short on time to keep it all off through physical activity, the Metabolic Breakthrough Nutrition Plan in combination with your activity program will see that you succeed and continue to keep it off.

Super Booster Program

A 15-minute walk (or equivalent *moderate* activity such as rebounding) after meals has proved to be the very best way to facilitate weight loss in the most difficult cases I have worked with. These most difficult cases are usually persons who are more than 50 pounds overweight and not in condition to move briskly enough, or for long enough at a brisk pace, to take full advantage of the calorie burning that continues to occur for hours after the completion of vigorous activity.

You will begin with one walk or some other moderate activity after your largest meal, and add other 15-minute periods after meals as the weeks progress. By the third week you will be able to substitute one *brisk* 30-minute activity period at Metabolic Improvement Intensity before dinner, if you choose. By the fourth week, you will have a choice of three alternatives:

1. moderate activity after meals or
2. combining a moderate activity after your largest meal with *brisk* activity before dinner or
3. getting in a full 45 minutes of *brisk* activity before dinner.

All activity is done at a moderate pace after meals, or builds to a brisk pace before dinner, as in the regular program. If your weight loss is satisfactory, switch over to either the regular or the advanced program whenever you please.

Strict adherence to the Super Booster schedule—activity after meals or just before dinner—for one month will stimulate the most stubborn metabolisms. At the end of that time, you will have lost considerable weight and made some major changes in your metabolic processes. You can then be more flexible.

I know you are wondering which is better—the moderate after-meal activity or the brisk prolonged activity. Unfortunately, there is no controlled research to indicate which is the better choice in any given instance. Almost everyone prefers to switch into more brisk, prolonged activity as soon as they are capable of it. I think you will, too. It is psychologically more satisfying. However, in several instances with persons in the Vanderbilt program, for reasons I at this point do not understand, *nothing* worked as well to facilitate weight loss as walking after meals. All of these persons were very heavy and lifelong dieters.

Most persons can walk at a comfortable pace soon after eating without noticing any ill effects. However, when you first begin the program I think it is advisable to test your body's reactions and wait about 20 minutes after your meals. This is especially important if you are considerably overweight and walking at any time feels effortful. If you experience no ill effects, feel free to walk as soon as you like. Discontinue walking if you experience any gastric distress or shortness of breath at what is normally your most comfortable pace.

Advanced Program

If you have been active once or twice a week in a regular exercise class or an active sport, you are way ahead of the game. You can start right out at a much higher level. Test yourself with a brisk 15- or 30-minute walk on Day 1, and proceed to build to the full 45 minutes of *brisk* activity at Metabolic Breakthrough Intensity as soon as you can without injury to your weight-bearing joints and muscles. Examine the suggested schedules in Table 13-1 and at the start of each week of the 28-day program.

TABLE 13-1
28-Day Metabolic Breakthrough Activity Program

Regular Program

WEEK 1

Goal 15 minutes daily of whole-body movement activity.
Less than 50 pounds overweight: moderate tempo (in walking, approximately 3 MPH)
More than 50 pounds overweight: slow tempo (in walking, less than 3 MPH)
Activity can be broken up into 5-minute periods, if necessary.

WEEK 2

Goal 15 minutes of daily activity at *Metabolic Breakthrough Intensity* (70 to 90 percent of maximum heart rate).
Less than 50 pounds overweight: brisk tempo (in walking, 3.5 to 4.5 MPH)
More than 50 pounds overweight: moderate tempo (in walking, approximately 3 MPH)
Heavier persons reach metabolic breakthrough intensity at a slower pace than lighter persons.
Activity can be broken up into 5-minute periods, if necessary.

TABLE 13-1 *(Continued)*

WEEK 3

Goal   30 minutes of daily activity at *Metabolic Breakthrough Intensity*.

Adjust the pace or tempo of activity to reach 70 to 90 percent of your maximum heart rate, or simply use the perceived effort that corresponds to *brisk* activity as your guide.

Activity can be broken up into shorter periods. However, a full 30 minutes at a single stretch is generally required to obtain continued calorie-burning effects for hours after the conclusion of activity.

WEEK 4

Goal   45 minutes of daily activity at *Metabolic Breakthrough Intensity*.

Adjust the pace or tempo of activity to reach 70 to 90 percent of your maximum heart rate, or simply use the perceived effort that corresponds to *brisk* activity as your guide.

Activity can be broken up into shorter periods. However, a full 30 minutes at a single stretch is generally required to obtain continued calorie-burning effects for hours after the conclusion of activity.

You have reached the final goal: each day's activity burns enough calories to keep approximately 50 pounds of fat off your body after you reach desired weight.

Super Booster Program

The Super Booster Program is designed to facilitate weight loss in persons who have difficulty losing weight on anything other than semi-starvation diet plans. It must be followed as long as weight loss does not proceed at a rate of from 1 to 3 pounds per week on the Regular Program. As soon as your rate of loss reaches that level, you may switch to a more flexible activity schedule.

WEEK 1

Goal   15 minutes of whole-body movement activity *done at your naturally occurring daily metabolic high points.*

Less than 50 pounds overweight: A single block of moderately paced walking (3 MPH) or rebounding for 15 minutes after your largest meal.

More than 50 pounds overweight: A single block of slow-paced walking (under 3 MPH) or gentle rebounding for 15 minutes after your largest meal.

(Be sure to read my recommendations on pp. 83–85 for walking after meals.)

TABLE 13-1 *(Continued)*

WEEK 2

Goal 15 minutes of whole-body movement activity *done at your naturally occurring daily metabolic high points.*

Less than 50 pounds overweight: moderate activity after your largest meal as in Week 1, or *brisk* activity, done at *Metabolic Breakthrough Intensity* (70 to 90 percent of your maximum heart rate) before dinner.

More than 50 pounds overweight: gentle activity after your largest meal, as in Week 1, or *moderate* activity before dinner. You will reach Metabolic Breakthrough Intensity at a more moderate pace because of your added weight.

WEEK 3

Goal 30 minutes of whole-body movement activity *done at your naturally occurring daily metabolic high points.*
1. two 15-minute activity sessions after meals or
2. one 15-minute session after your largest meal and a *brisk* 15-minute session, at *Metabolic Breakthrough Intensity,* before dinner or
3. a single, *brisk* 30-minute session before dinner.

Persons more than 50 pounds overweight will reach Metabolic Breakthrough Intensity with moderately paced activity.

WEEK 4

Goal 45 minutes of whole-body movement activity *done at your naturally occurring daily metabolic high points.*
1. three 15-minute sessions after meals or
2. one 15-minute session after your largest meal and one *brisk* 30-minute session before dinner or
3. a single, *brisk* session of 45 minutes before dinner.

This week you reach the final goal: each day's activity burns enough calories to keep approximately 50 pounds of fat off your body when you reach desired weight.

Advanced Program

Persons less than 50 pounds overweight who have been involved in moderate activity at least once a week can begin with the Advanced Program and reach their fat-burning goal of 45 minutes of *brisk* activity each day as soon as possible. You must be the judge of your own condition, but discretion is the better part of valor! It is better to reach your goal a few days later than to injure yourself in your enthusiasm and delay it for several weeks.

TABLE 13-1 *(Continued)*

WEEK 1

Goal 15 to 30 minutes of *brisk* whole-body movement *(Metabolic Breakthrough Intensity, 70 to 90 percent of your maximum heart rate)*.

Any combination of 5-, 10-, or 15-minute segments, or a single 30-minute session.

It takes 30 minutes at Metabolic Breakthrough Intensity to obtain prolonged calorie-burning benefits after the completion of activity.

WEEK 2

Goal 30 to 45 minutes of *brisk* whole-body movement *(Metabolic Breakthrough Intensity as above)*.

Any combination of 5-, 10-, 15-, or 30-minute segments, or a single 45-minute session.

WEEK 3

Goal 45 minutes of *brisk* whole-body movement, as above.

Any combination of time periods, but remember that it takes at least 30 minutes at *Metabolic Breakthrough Intensity* to obtain those prolonged calorie-burning benefits.

When you reach 45 minutes of whole-body movement physical activity, you reach the ultimate goal of the 28-Day Metabolic Breakthrough Activity Program: you are burning enough calories to keep approximately 50 pounds of fat off your body once you reach your desired weight.

WEEK 4

You reached your goal in Week 3. Continue with your program, or aim for a single session of 45 minutes each day. That will provide the maximum metabolic improvement returns for the effort you invest.

14

THE 28-DAY METABOLIC BREAKTHROUGH NUTRITION PLAN

The 28-Day Nutrition Plan is based on United States Senate Select Committee recommendations for percentages of carbohydrate, protein, and fat in the diet (approximately 60, 15, and 25 percent, respectively). It is also designed to meet the Recommended Dietary Allowances (RDAs) established by the Food and Nutrition Board of the National Research Council.

However, the 28-Day Metabolic Breakthrough Nutrition Plan goes beyond these recommendations in the way it orders and combines foods.

There is a specific menu (beginning on p. 105) for each of the 28 days that maximizes the metabolic benefits of the AC/DC ratio. Page numbers for recipes are given in parentheses. Each meal contains at least two foods high in dietary fiber to aid intestinal motility and prevent the absorption of a certain amount of the fat you will still use for flavor and satiety value. Snacks are always chosen from high-fiber fruits and vegetables. By eating AC foods at every meal and for snacks, you will tend to keep your metabolic rate higher than if you had eaten the same number of calories from foods in the DC category.

The Nutrition Plan also suggests that you move some of your food intake up to an earlier time of day if you have been skipping breakfast and a mid-morning snack. Remember that you burn more of the calories in your food in the process of digestion earlier in the day than later. Nevertheless, the meal plan is a compromise with our usual eating habits, and all evening meals are designed so that you can still enjoy dinners with your family without having to prepare special foods for yourself.

When you use standard restaurant-size portions, a woman's daily food intake will be between 1200 and 1300 calories. When you follow the AC/DC ratio, you are assured of obtaining the nutrients contained in a wide variety of grains, fruits, and vegetables. Women need approximately 6 ounces of lean meat, fish, or fowl (cooked weight) each day for protein. Think in terms of two 3-ounce servings if you like to have a meat dish twice a day. You do not need to eat meat, however, in order to obtain high-quality protein. You can obtain the equivalent from complementary protein foods (grains, legumes, nuts, and seeds in combination) such as are illustrated in the vegetarian dishes contained in a number of the daily menus. Adding a small amount of a milk product, such as cheese or yogurt, also greatly increases the quality of protein obtained from plant sources.

Women should be careful to eat two servings of food high in calcium each day. I emphasize this need because studies show that women's diets frequently are deficient in calcium. I see it each year in the eating diaries kept for me by students in one of my undergraduate seminars. The shortage occurs in part because of a poor choice of foods, and in part because women don't consume as much food as men and therefore don't have the opportunity to obtain the small amounts of calcium that occur in vegetables and whole grains. Because of this deficiency, women suffer from far more bone fractures later in life than men. The bone deterioration that seems to be occurring as we grow older really has its start in our thirties, in part because of this dietary deficiency, and in part because of a lack of exercise. The deterioration may be accelerated after menopause, due to hormone changes, but it can be remedied to a large extent by proper diet and adequate exercise. Milk and milk products, other than butter, and canned sardines or salmon that still have the bones are excellent sources of calcium. You can also obtain a significant amount of calcium by chewing the ends of chicken bones.

Men should use portions that are approximately 50 percent larger than women, concentrating on increasing fruits, vegetables, and whole grains. Men's protein needs can be met with 9 to 10 ounces of lean meat, fish, or fowl (two 4.5- to 5-ounce servings) as well as with the equivalent in complementary protein dishes. Men should also have a minimum of two servings of foods rich in calcium each day. With these suggestions men will be obtaining a daily intake of about 1800 calories. By combining this Nutrition Plan with the Breakthrough Activity Program, you should easily achieve a weight loss of 2 or more pounds per week.

Drink plenty of water, at least eight glasses per day. In addition to helping prevent water retention and stimulating kidney action, water adds to the volume that your digestive system has to process without adding calories. It speeds up your metabolism. By drinking a glass of water before and after each meal, and one more glass of water with your mid-morning and mid-afternoon snacks, you will be giving your system a very healthy workout and it will burn an even larger number of extra calories. Save room to drink water *after* as well as before meals. Plan for this, since it means you will have to stop eating before you reach the satiation point with food, and have a glass of water instead. In addition, keep a glass of water handy throughout the day (iced, with a slice of lemon or lime in it is very refreshing). *The more water you drink, the faster you will lose weight.*

The Daily Menu and Eating Record

Every day's nutrition plan is presented in two ways to allow for utmost convenience and flexibility. A specific menu appears to the left on each page of the daily plan (pp. 105–35). And what an adventure in gourmet eating it is! It features an international cuisine through which I demonstrate that you can eat in any style you wish —French, Italian, German, Indian, Mexican, just name it—and still apply the AC/DC ratio and keep your fats and processed foods at the levels our leading nutritionists recommend.

But there is no need to be rigid. You are not required to follow my daily menus exactly if any particular dish doesn't appeal to your taste or if your family is not quite ready to be so adventurous. At the beginning of my recipe section (pp. 153–206) you will find easy-to-use Food Exchange and Calorie Counter Lists. Feel free to use fruits, vegetables, and grains interchangeably, always being sure that you choose from a wide variety throughout the week. You can substitute meat, fish, or fowl from the Exchange List and use any of your present favorite recipes modified according to the guidelines for reducing fat and sugar given at the beginning of the recipe section. You can also substitute more of my complementary protein vegetarian dishes for meat dishes.

You can use foods from the Milk List interchangeably, substituting low-fat milk or yogurt for cheese, or vice versa. Note that many varieties of cheese contain a large amount of fat as well as calcium, so it is not a good idea to exceed the recommended two servings if you use cheese as your primary source of calcium.

However, this flexibility, which allows you to adapt the program to suit your food preferences, *does not give you license to deviate from the principles of the basic nutrition plan.* If you do, you will slow your rate of weight loss. You *must* implement the AC/DC ratio, have two servings of a high-fiber food with each meal, and use only high-fiber snacks to obtain maximum metabolic benefits. The AC group of foods is located together in the Exchange Lists.

The Exchange Lists also contain the most up-to-date fiber content information on various foods, as well as the calories. If you wish to keep track of your fiber count, approximately 30 grams per day, give or take a few, is considered a healthy amount. If you go as high as 50, you may be bothered by excessive gas, so I would advise you not to overdo it.

In order to be sure that you are obtaining adequate nutrition and implementing the program correctly, a shorthand record form is presented on the right side of each day's plan. Directions for its use are given in Chapter 15 and an illustration appears on page 99.

The Perfect-Day Dessert

Each day's menu concludes with a *Perfect-Day Dessert.* It's called the "perfect-day dessert" because your choice of food when you finish the day can contribute a great deal to whether or not you are implementing the Nutrition Plan correctly.

At dinnertime each day, use of the shorthand record form next to the day's menu will give you an opportunity to review your nutrition plan to see whether you have fulfilled the requirements of the AC/DC ratio and your body's need for calcium (two servings) and protein (two servings). You can then make a choice with respect to that second DC allowance.

If you have gotten your eight servings of foods from the AC list, and have avoided fatty foods, your Perfect-Day Dessert might be selected from one of my own dessert recipes (p. 198) to round out that "2" part of your 8/2 AC/DC ratio. There is no need to deny yourself a serving of delicious Peach or Blueberry Kuchen (p. 199) or even Cheese Pie (p. 200) when you follow the 28-Day Metabolic Breakthrough Nutrition Plan and Activity Program. But be sure to choose fruit or fruit and cheese for that dessert if you have not gotten your eight AC servings during the day or your two servings of foods high in calcium.

Basic Substitutions

Because making substitutions creates problems for so many people, I have prepared some Basic Substitution Meals that can always be used.

These Basic Substitutions are designed to make your Nutrition Plan as simple as possible. You can use them as often as you like.

Your entire 28-Day Metabolic Breakthrough Nutrition Plan can be composed of these three meals and you would be assured of adequate nutrition as well as weight loss.

Whenever you do find that one of my suggestions does not appeal to you, or whenever you are too busy to plan your own substitutions, these should be your meals. They are simple and satisfying, they relieve you of the need to make any decisions, and you will never be hungry.

Basic Breakfast

2 slices whole-wheat bread
2 ounces your favorite cheese
Beverage
or
Cereal with milk
Beverage

Basic Lunch Substitution

Fresh fruit, whole or sliced, as much as you like
½ cup cottage cheese
2 T. chopped nuts

If you use this luncheon substitution at home, make it attractive by serving it over fresh greens.

If you will carry it to work and you do not have a means of refrigeration, put the cheese together with the cold fruit in a plastic container, double-bag it in plain brown paper bags, and it will stay cool for several hours.

If you don't care for cottage cheese, use hard cheese, or leave it out completely.

When I say "unlimited fruit" I really mean it—up to a point. My own bag might contain two apples, an orange or peach, and a banana. If you can eat more than that, you've exceeded my point!

Basic Dinner

6 to 9 ounces of lean meat, fish, or fowl, baked or broiled
Unlimited vegetables (from List I, p. 140)
Have at least one vegetable raw, or have a salad
Use your fat allowance for cooking and flavoring
One whole grapefruit, or two oranges, sectioned
(or substitute other fruit, different from your lunch selection)

I have given this menu to many busy people who have neither the time to fuss nor the desire to ever feel hungry. It has an excellent effect on your intestinal functions. Many people who have suffered lifelong problems with constipation, or who only experience a problem when they reduce calories, report that the grapefruit after dinner seems to be a sure formula for regularity.

The grapefruit after dinner is also your assurance that you will never go to bed hungry—you can have two if you like!

The above meal plan is almost exactly what I used every day for three to four weeks each time I cut calories on my way to a permanent 75-pound weight loss.

The only exceptions I made were when I ate out.

Now I'll show you how to do that, too.

Eating Out Meals

Dinner Out

Avoid rich sauces and choose plain food. If you don't know how to make the correct choice from an unusual selection, always revert to this good old standby:

Green salad, dressing on the side, use ½ T.
Broiled or baked fish, fowl, or lean meat
One or two vegetables
Baked potato with one pat of butter or 2 T. sour cream
Fresh fruit (ask for it)
     or
Roll you didn't eat before dinner
Beverage

If you cannot get fresh fruit, ask the waiter to bring you the roll you didn't eat before dinner, and have that with coffee while your friends are having a dessert. Plain bread goes very well with coffee after a meal, and it's very satisfying.

Lunch Out

So many restaurants have designed dishes for the calorie conscious that you shouldn't have any problem. But if you can't find a restaurant that has something special, here are your best choices from among the standard fare:

Bowl of soup, with slice of bread or half a dozen crackers
     or
Green salad, with an ounce each of cheese and ham
     or
Fresh fruit salad, with nuts or cheese
     or
The perennial dieter's special:
Lean beef patty, cottage cheese, coleslaw (or small salad)

Do not vary from the 28-Day Plan and you will lose weight. For me, using the type of menu I just described above, it was worth between 15 and 20 pounds a month of *real fat* loss, not water or lean muscle mass, each time I used it. And I never suffered a rebound weight gain as an aftermath.

Survey the Whole Program before You Begin

Before you begin your 28-Day Program, study the sample record described in Chapter 15, look over the record forms and menus, study the recipes, and examine the Exchange Lists (pp. 138–42). Decide which recipes you will use, and what foods you will need in order to make substitutions whenever you choose. Then, write out your shopping list and make sure you have everything you need for what I hope will be the tastiest and most satisfying nutrition plan you have ever followed.

15

KEEPING TRACK OF YOUR PROGRESS

On page 99 you will find a sample first day of a typical record. Across the top the woman in my example recorded the day number of her record, the date, and her weight. Since it was the first day there was no weight loss yet to be reported.

Under the heading "Metabolic Breakthrough Activity Program" she entered her Activity Goal of 15 minutes of walking and recorded, at the end of the day, that she walked 15 minutes at 5 P.M. (before dinner). She place a checkmark on the "yes" blank to indicate that her goal was reached and noted that she felt fine after her walk. Be sure to make whatever comments seem appropriate to the day's activities, since a review of your weight-loss progress, together with your comments, may give you some special insight as to the way your body responds to your activity and nutrition changes.

Her record under the heading "Metabolic Breakthrough Nutrition Plan" indicated that she made a few substitutions in the menu. She took a tuna sandwich with her to work, together with a packet of carrot and celery sticks, which she split up and had at lunch and for her afternoon snack. She followed the rest of the menu exactly, and noted her actual choice of fruits at breakfast, mid-morning, and dinner. She used her allowance of fat (which equals 3 teaspoons of butter, margarine, or oil) in part on her sandwich and in part for cooking the evening meal.

In order to be sure that her diet contained the recommended servings in each of the food groups, she placed a slash mark (/) for each serving of food that she actually consumed on the lines provided in the Eating Record on the lower right portion of the page. Before choosing her dessert for dinner, she followed the direction to "check eating record" in the Menu, and noted that only one slash mark appeared on the Milk Group line. This mark represented the milk that she had for breakfast. Thus, she chose an apple and cheese for dessert, and placed the second slash mark on the Milk Group line, as well as another on the Fruits line under the AC Group heading. She then totaled her marks in the AC and DC categories, and you can see that her AC/DC ratio ended up at 9/1. That's even better than the minimum standard of 8/1 or 8/2 required by the plan. The more AC for DC substitutions you make, the better.

Finally—and this is very important—notice also that she checked "yes" on the line "Eight glasses of water?" Those eight glasses of water, with meals and snacks, helped keep her metabolism chugging along, burning extra calories all day long.

Make sure your record looks like the one on the next page and you will be off to an excellent start.

Keeping Your Own Record

Record forms for your own 28-Day Metabolic Breakthrough Program, arranged in four weekly sets, begin on page 104.

The first two pages are your overall MASTER RECORD of weight and body dimension changes that will occur during the 28 days, with instructions on how to obtain these measurements preceding the forms. You will record your weight first thing upon arising each day on the 28-day plan, but enter on the MASTER RECORD the weights for Days 1, 8, 15, 22, and 29 so that you can observe your progress by the week.

Take your body measurements on these same five MASTER RECORD days, according to the directions given.

If you have a good imagination, you can play an interesting mental game with these lost inches. It goes like this:

If you were able to take all the fat you will lose and put it into a single cylinder about 2½ feet high, that cylinder would have a circumference just about equal to the total inches you will lose in your body measurements. It gets amazingly large if you have more than a few pounds to lose.

For example, while losing about 30 pounds, women will lose

Day _____1_____   Date _6/1/83_   Weight _170_ lbs.

24-hour change ___—___ lbs.   Total loss _—_ lbs.

Metabolic Breakthrough Activity Program

Activity Goal _15 min. walking_

ACTIVITY RECORD

Kind of Activity	Amount	Time of Day
Walking	15 min	5:00 PM

Goal Reached ___✓___ (yes) _____ (no)

Comments:
Felt fine

Metabolic Breakthrough Nutrition Plan

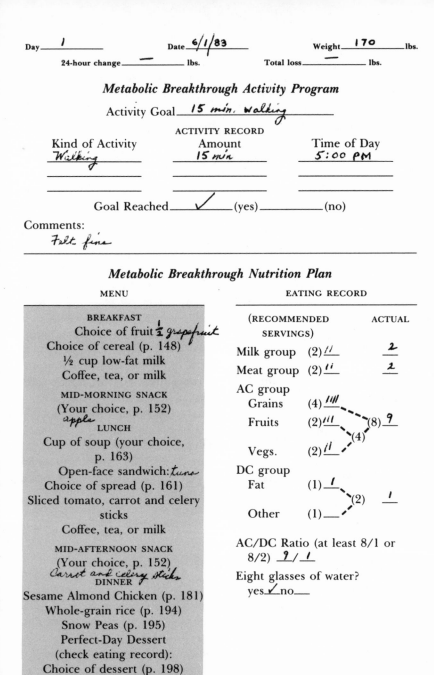

MENU

BREAKFAST
Choice of fruit ½ grapefruit
Choice of cereal (p. 148)
½ cup low-fat milk
Coffee, tea, or milk

MID-MORNING SNACK
(Your choice, p. 152)
apple
LUNCH
Cup of soup (your choice, p. 163)
Open-face sandwich: tuna
Choice of spread (p. 161)
Sliced tomato, carrot and celery sticks
Coffee, tea, or milk

MID-AFTERNOON SNACK
(Your choice, p. 152)
Carrot and celery sticks
DINNER
Sesame Almond Chicken (p. 181)
Whole-grain rice (p. 194)
Snow Peas (p. 195)
Perfect-Day Dessert
(check eating record):
Choice of dessert (p. 198)
or
apple Fruit and cheese 1 oz.
Beverage

EATING RECORD

(RECOMMENDED SERVINGS)		ACTUAL
Milk group	(2) //	2
Meat group	(2) //	2
AC group		
Grains	(4) ////	
Fruits	(2) ///	(8) 9
	(4)	
Vegs.	(2) //	
DC group		
Fat	(1) /	
	(2)	1
Other	(1)	

AC/DC Ratio (at least 8/1 or 8/2) _9_/_1_

Eight glasses of water?
yes ✓ no ___

99

about 20 inches in the parts of the body you will be measuring. That 20 inches represents a column of fat stretching from your knees to your chin with a 20-inch circumference, or a diameter of about 7 inches. *Now, that's a lot of fat!*

Continue as follows:

1. At the start of each week is a cover sheet summarizing the goals of each of the three levels of the Metabolic Breakthrough Activity Program. Decide on your personal level. You may proceed from the Regular Program to the Advanced Program more quickly if you find that you respond without any adverse effects to the lower level of exercise. And you can experiment with the Super Booster Program if weight comes off slowly and you want to speed your losses.

2. Four sets of seven daily recording sheets follow. Enter your Activity Goal for the day and be sure to check off "Goal Reached ___(yes)" each day!

3. Sample the featured dishes each week to expand your awareness of different styles of nutritious food preparation, or make appropriate substitutions when necessary. However, be sure you note any substitutions that you make in the Nutrition Plan, and make your substitutions from the equivalent Exchange Lists, using low-fat and low-sugar recipes. *Always total your AC/DC ratio*—an 8/2 or 8/1 ratio (you can go higher on the AC side) forms the basis of one of the most important changes you will be making in the quality of your nutrition. Assuming an adequate intake of calcium and protein foods, the AC/DC ratio assures that you will be doing everything it takes from the nutritional side of the Metabolic Breakthrough Plan to achieve permanent weight control, as well as all-around good health.

Directions for Using the Master Record Form

The Master Record Form offers a convenient way to keep track of your weight-loss and body circumference changes.

Enter your weight at the beginning of the program and each week, according to the directions on the form.

Take your body circumference measurements on the upper right arm, chest, waist, hips, and upper right thigh. These are representative of your major fat deposits. Be sure to take the measurements

at the points located in the diagram below:
    Upper right arm at its largest circumference
    Chest at its largest circumference
    Waist about 1 inch above the navel
    Hips at their widest point
    Thigh high near the crotch, at its largest circumference
    Be sure to take the measurements at the same points each time.
Let your measuring tape fit snugly around your body, but *do not squeeze!* Apply the same pressure each time you take a measurement.

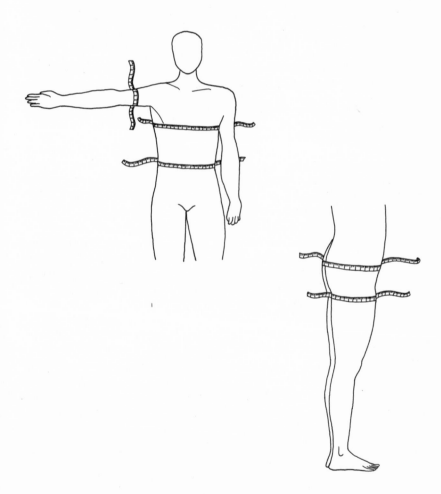

Master Record Form

Summary of Weight Loss

Enter your starting weight on Day 1, and then your weight on Days 8, 15, 22, and 29 from the Daily Records that follow. Each week, subtract your weight from the week before, and enter that week's loss. Total the loss over four weeks.

Initial Weight Day 1 _____lbs.

      Weight Day 8 _____lbs.   _____Lbs. Lost in Week 1

      Weight Day 15 _____lbs.   _____Lbs. Lost in Week 2

      Weight Day 22 _____lbs.   _____Lbs. Lost in Week 3

      Weight Day 29 _____lbs.   _____Lbs. Lost in Week 4

                            _____Total Weight Loss

Body Circumference Changes

Take your body circumference measurements each week, according to the directions on pages 100–101. Enter your initial measurements on Day 1, and then the measurements on Days 8, 15, 22, and 29. Each week, subtract the new measurement from the one you obtained the week before. Total the loss over four weeks.

UPPER RIGHT ARM

Day 1 __ In.
Day 8 __ In. __ In. Lost Wk. 1
Day 15 __ In. __ In. Lost Wk. 2
Day 22 __ In. __ In. Lost Wk. 3
Day 29 __ In. __ In. Lost Wk. 4
          __ Total In. Lost

CHEST

Day 1 __ In.
Day 8 __ In. __ In. Lost Wk. 1
Day 15 __ In. __ In. Lost Wk. 2
Day 22 __ In. __ In. Lost Wk. 3
Day 29 __ In. __ In. Lost Wk. 4
          __ Total In. Lost

WAIST

Day 1 __ In.
Day 8 __ In. __ In. Lost Wk. 1
Day 15 __ In. __ In. Lost Wk. 2
Day 22 __ In. __ In. Lost Wk. 3
Day 29 __ In. __ In. Lost Wk. 4
          __ Total In. Lost

HIPS

Day 1 __ In.
Day 8 __ In. __ In. Lost Wk. 1
Day 15 __ In. __ In. Lost Wk. 2
Day 22 __ In. __ In. Lost Wk. 3
Day 29 __ In. __ In. Lost Wk. 4
          __ Total In. Lost

UPPER RIGHT THIGH

Day 1 ___ In.
Day 8 ___ In. ___ In. Lost Wk. 1
Day 15 ___ In. ___ In. Lost Wk. 2
Day 22 ___ In. ___ In. Lost Wk. 3
Day 29 ___ In. ___ In. Lost Wk. 4

___ Total In. Lost

Weekly Summary of Body Circumference Changes

Take the amount you have lost each week in each of your body circumference measurements and enter it on the appropriate line below. Then total up the losses for each week.

INCHES LOST:	WEEK 1	WEEK 2	WEEK 3	WEEK 4
Upper Arm	_____	_____	_____	_____
Chest	_____	_____	_____	_____
Waist	_____	_____	_____	_____
Hips	_____	_____	_____	_____
Thigh	_____	_____	_____	_____
Totals	_____	_____	_____	_____

Program Summary of Body Circumference Changes

Combine the total number of inches you have lost each week in all the body measurements above and enter the totals at the end of your 28-Day Metabolic Breakthrough Program in the summary table below.

TOTAL INCHES LOST

Week 1 _____
Week 2 _____
Week 3 _____
Week 4 _____

_____ Grand Total All Inches Lost

DIRECTIONS

WEEK 1

I. Enter day number, date, weight, 24-hour change, and total weight lost since the start of the program.

II. Daily Metabolic Breakthrough Activity Program

A. *Regular Program* 15 minutes of activity (whole-body movement), moderate pace, done at any convenient time, in any combination of 5-, 10-, or a single 15-minute period.

B. *Super Booster Program* 15 minutes of activity (whole-body movement) done after your largest meal, or in the late afternoon. If you are not in shape to do the equivalent of walking for a continuous 15 minutes, build up to it gradually until you reach it at the end of the week.

C. *Advanced Program* 15 to 30 minutes of *brisk* activity (whole-body movement) in any combination of 5-, 10-, or 15-minute segments, or a single 30-minute segment.

III. Daily Metabolic Breakthrough Nutrition Plan

A. Follow the menus exactly or make appropriate substitutions, filling in the food record in the lower right portion of each page.

B. This week's menu features the following dinner recipes from the Metabolic Breakthrough Nutrition Plan:
1. Sesame Almond Chicken (Oriental Style) p. 181.
2. Cheddar Chile Pie (Mexican) p. 175.
3. Fillet of Sole Florentine (Italian) p. 178.
4. Marinated Flank Steak (a choice of marinades) p. 179.
5. Lemon-Baked Chicken (American) p. 179.
6. Spinach Pesto and Pasta (Vegetarian, Italian) p. 184.
7. Oven-Fried Catfish (Southern) p. 180.

Day_____ Date_____ Weight_____lbs.

24-hour change_____ lbs. Total loss_____ lbs.

Metabolic Breakthrough Activity Program

Activity Goal_____

ACTIVITY RECORD

Kind of Activity	Amount	Time of Day
_____	_____	_____
_____	_____	_____
_____	_____	_____

Goal Reached_____(yes)_____(no)

Comments:

Metabolic Breakthrough Nutrition Plan

MENU	EATING RECORD

MENU

BREAKFAST
Choice of fruit
Choice of cereal (pp. 148–49)
½ cup low-fat milk
Coffee, tea, or milk

MID-MORNING SNACK
(Your choice, p. 152)

LUNCH
Cup of soup (your choice, p. 163)
Open-face sandwich:
Choice of spread (p. 161)
Sliced tomato, carrot and celery
sticks
Coffee, tea, or milk

MID-AFTERNOON SNACK
(Your choice, p. 152)

DINNER
Sesame Almond Chicken (p. 181)
Whole-grain rice (p. 194)
Snow Peas (p. 195)
Perfect-Day Dessert
(check eating record):
Choice of dessert (p. 198)
or
Fruit and cheese
Beverage

EATING RECORD

(RECOMMENDED   ACTUAL
SERVINGS)

Milk group   (2)___   ___

Meat group   (2)___   ___

AC group
Grains   (4)___
Fruits   (2)___ (8)___
(4)
Vegs.   (2)___

DC group
Fat   (1)___
(2)   ___
Other   (1)___

AC/DC Ratio (at least 8/1 or
8/2) ___/___

Eight glasses of water?
yes___no___

Day_____ Date_____ Weight_____lbs.

24-hour change_____ lbs. Total loss_____ lbs.

Metabolic Breakthrough Activity Program

Activity Goal_____

Kind of Activity	Amount	Time of Day
_____	_____	_____
_____	_____	_____
_____	_____	_____

Goal Reached_____(yes)_____(no)

Comments:

Metabolic Breakthrough Nutrition Plan

MENU

BREAKFAST
2 slices whole-wheat
bread (p. 203)
1 T. peanut butter
(or favorite spread, p. 161)
Milk, tea, or coffee

MID-MORNING SNACK
(Your choice, p. 152)

LUNCH
Piquant Salad (p. 156)
White Wine Vinegar
Dressing (p. 160)
3 oz. sliced chicken or turkey
Milk, tea, or coffee

MID-AFTERNOON SNACK
(Your choice, p. 152)

DINNER
Cheddar Chile Pie (p. 175)
Cauliflower Casserole (p. 188)
Perfect-Day Dessert
(check eating record):
Choice of dessert (p. 198)
or
Fruit
Beverage

EATING RECORD

(RECOMMENDED   ACTUAL
SERVINGS)

Milk group (2)___   ___

Meat group (2)___   ___

AC group
  Grains (4)___
  Fruits (2)___ ‾(8)___
              (4)
  Vegs. (2)___

DC group
  Fat (1)___
            ‾(2)   ___
  Other (1)___

AC/DC Ratio (at least 8/1 or
8/2) ___/___

Eight glasses of water?
yes___no___

Day_____ Date_____ Weight_____lbs.

24-hour change_____ lbs. Total loss_____ lbs.

Metabolic Breakthrough Activity Program

Activity Goal_____

ACTIVITY RECORD

Kind of Activity	Amount	Time of Day
_____	_____	_____
_____	_____	_____
_____	_____	_____

Goal Reached_____(yes)_____(no)

Comments:

Metabolic Breakthrough Nutrition Plan

MENU

BREAKFAST
Choice of cereal (pp. 148–49)
½ cup low-fat milk
Coffee, tea, or milk

MID-MORNING SNACK
(Your choice, p. 152)

LUNCH
Creative Fruit Salad (p. 154)
½ cup low-fat cottage cheese
Coffee, tea, or milk

MID-AFTERNOON SNACK
(Your choice, p. 152)

DINNER
Fillet of Sole Florentine (p. 178)
Seasoned Tomatoes (p. 195)
Pennsylvania Dutch Potato
Pudding (p. 193)
Perfect-Day Dessert
(check eating record):
Choice of dessert (p. 198)
or
Fruit and cheese
Beverage

EATING RECORD

(RECOMMENDED   ACTUAL
SERVINGS)

Milk group   (2)__   __

Meat group   (2)__   __

AC group
  Grains   (4)__
  Fruits   (2)__   (8)__
          (4)
  Vegs.   (2)__

DC group
  Fat   (1)__
          (2)   __
  Other   (1)__

AC/DC Ratio (at least 8/1 or
8/2) __/__

Eight glasses of water?
yes__no__

Day_____ Date_____ Weight_____lbs.

24-hour change_____ lbs. Total loss_____ lbs.

Metabolic Breakthrough Activity Program

Activity Goal_____

ACTIVITY RECORD

Kind of Activity	Amount	Time of Day
_____	_____	_____
_____	_____	_____
_____	_____	_____

Goal Reached_____(yes)_____(no)

Comments:

Metabolic Breakthrough Nutrition Plan

MENU

BREAKFAST
Sliced orange
2 slices whole-wheat toast
2 oz. your favorite cheese
Milk, tea, or coffee

MID-MORNING SNACK
(Your choice, p. 152)

LUNCH
Tuna or Salmon Salad (p. 157)
on greens, with sliced tomatoes,
cucumbers, and radishes
Milk, tea, or coffee

MID-AFTERNOON SNACK
(Your choice, p. 152)

DINNER
Marinated Flank Steak (p. 179)
Stir-fry Spinach (or other greens,
p. 196)
Baked potato with
cottage cheese dressing (p. 161)
Perfect-Day Dessert
(check eating record):
Choice of dessert (p. 198)
or
Fruit
Beverage

EATING RECORD

	(RECOMMENDED SERVINGS)	ACTUAL
Milk group	(2)__	__
Meat group	(2)__	__
AC group		
Grains	(4)__	
Fruits	(2)__	(8)__
	(4)	
Vegs.	(2)__	
DC group		
Fat	(1)__	
	(2)	__
Other	(1)__	

AC/DC Ratio (at least 8/1 or
8/2) __/__

Eight glasses of water?
yes__no__

Day_____   Date_____   Weight_____lbs.

   24-hour change_____ lbs.   Total loss_____ lbs.

Metabolic Breakthrough Activity Program

Activity Goal_____

ACTIVITY RECORD

Kind of Activity	Amount	Time of Day
_____	_____	_____
_____	_____	_____
_____	_____	_____

Goal Reached_____(yes)_____(no)

Comments:

Metabolic Breakthrough Nutrition Plan

MENU	EATING RECORD

BREAKFAST
Choice of fruit
Choice of cereal (pp. 148–49)
½ cup low-fat milk
Coffee, tea, or milk

MID-MORNING SNACK
(Your choice, p. 152)

LUNCH
Creative Chef Salad (p. 154)
Choice of dressing (p. 158)
1 slice whole-wheat bread
or 4 crackers
Coffee, tea, or milk

MID-AFTERNOON SNACK
(Your choice, p. 152)

DINNER
Lemon-Baked Chicken (p. 179)
Chana Aur Aloo
(Indian chickpeas and
potatoes, p. 190)
Green vegetable (p. 196)
Perfect-Day Dessert
(check eating record):
Choice of dessert (p. 198)
or
Fruit and cheese
Beverage

(RECOMMENDED   ACTUAL
   SERVINGS)

Milk group   (2)__   __

Meat group   (2)__   __

AC group
   Grains   (4)__
   Fruits   (2)__   (8)__
                    (4)
   Vegs.   (2)__

DC group
   Fat   (1)__
                    (2)   __
   Other   (1)__

AC/DC Ratio (at least 8/1 or
8/2) __/__

Eight glasses of water?
yes__no__

Day_____ Date_____ Weight_____lbs.

24-hour change_____ lbs. Total loss_____ lbs.

Metabolic Breakthrough Activity Program

Activity Goal_____

ACTIVITY RECORD

Kind of Activity	Amount	Time of Day
_____	_____	_____
_____	_____	_____
_____	_____	_____

Goal Reached_____(yes)_____(no)

Comments:

Metabolic Breakthrough Nutrition Plan

MENU   EATING RECORD

BREAKFAST
Try this for variety:
Choice of fruit
3 oz. lean beef patty
on 1 slice whole-wheat
toast (or use a basic
breakfast)
Milk, tea, or coffee

MID-MORNING SNACK
(Your choice, p. 152)

LUNCH
Seafood Soup Creole (p. 168)
1 slice whole-wheat bread or
4 crackers
Assorted raw vegetables, List I
(p. 140)
Milk, tea, or coffee

MID-AFTERNOON SNACK
(Your choice, p. 152)

DINNER
Spinach Pesto and Pasta (p. 184)
Tossed salad (p. 157)
Choice of dressing (p. 158)
Perfect-Day Dessert
(check eating record):
Choice of dessert
or
Fruit and 2 oz. cheese
Beverage

(RECOMMENDED   ACTUAL
SERVINGS)

Milk group (2)___   ___

Meat group (2)___   ___

AC group
Grains (4)___
Fruits (2)___ ___(8)___
(4)
Vegs. (2)___

DC group
Fat (1)___
(2) ___
Other (1)___

AC/DC Ratio (at least 8/1 or
8/2) ___/___

Eight glasses of water?
yes___no___

Day_____   Date_____   Weight_____lbs.

24-hour change_____ lbs.   Total loss_____ lbs.

Metabolic Breakthrough Activity Program

Activity Goal_____

ACTIVITY RECORD

Kind of Activity	Amount	Time of Day
_____	_____	_____
_____	_____	_____
_____	_____	_____

Goal Reached_____(yes)_____(no)

Comments:

Metabolic Breakthrough Nutrition Plan

MENU   EATING RECORD

BREAKFAST
½ grapefruit or melon
1 slice whole-wheat bread
1 t. your favorite preserves
Milk, tea, or coffee

MID-MORNING SNACK
(Your choice, p. 152)

LUNCH
Ratatouille
(hot or cold vegetables, p. 194)
2 slices whole-wheat bread
1 oz. hard cheese or grated
for salad
Milk, tea, or coffee

MID-AFTERNOON SNACK
(Your choice, p. 152)

DINNER
Oven-Fried Catfish (p. 180)
Oven-Fried Potato Sticks (p. 192)
Tossed salad (p. 157)
Choice of dressing (p. 158)
Perfect-Day Dessert
(check eating record):
Choice of dessert (p. 198)
or
Fruit and cheese
Beverage

(RECOMMENDED   ACTUAL
    SERVINGS)

Milk group   (2) ___   ___

Meat group (2) ___   ___

AC group
    Grains   (4) ___
    Fruits   (2) ___   (8) ___
                    (4)
    Vegs.   (2) ___

DC group
    Fat   (1) ___
                    (2)   ___
    Other   (1) ___

AC/DC Ratio (at least 8/1 or
8/2) ___/___

Eight glasses of water?
yes___no___

DIRECTIONS

WEEK 2

I. Enter day number, date, weight, 24-hour change, and total weight lost since the start of the program.

II. Daily Metabolic Breakthrough Activity Program

   A. *Regular Program* 15 minutes of activity (whole-body movement), *brisk* pace, done at any convenient time, in any combination of 5-, 10-, or a single 15-minute period.
   B. *Super Booster Program* 15 minutes of activity (whole-body movement), *moderate pace* if done after your largest meal, or in the late afternoon *at a brisk pace.*
   C. *Advanced Program* 30 to 45 minutes of *brisk* activity (whole-body movement) in any combination of 5-, 10-, 15-, or 30-minute segments, or a single 45-minute segment.

III. Daily Metabolic Breakthrough Nutrition Plan

   A. Follow the menus exactly or make appropriate substitutions, filling in the food record in the lower right portion of each page.
   B. This week's menu features the following recipes from the Metabolic Breakthrough Nutrition Plan:
      1. Chicken with Broccoli (Oriental) p. 176.
      2. Cabbage Rolls (German) p. 174.
      3. Fish Roll-ups (Italian/Jewish) p. 178.
      4. Baked Pork Chops (Middle European) p. 172.
      5. Spicy Chicken (East Indian) p. 183.
      6. Spaghetti w/Garlic and Clam Sauce (Italian) p. 182.
      7. Crab Quiche w/Crumb Topping (French) p. 176.

Metabolic Breakthrough Activity Program

Activity Goal_____

ACTIVITY RECORD

Kind of Activity	Amount	Time of Day
_____	_____	_____
_____	_____	_____
_____	_____	_____

Goal Reached_____(yes)_____(no)

Comments:

Metabolic Breakthrough Nutrition Plan

MENU   EATING RECORD

BREAKFAST
Choice of fruit
2 slices whole-wheat bread
1 T. peanut butter
(or favorite spread, p. 161)
Milk, tea, or coffee

MID-MORNING SNACK
(Your choice, p. 152)

LUNCH
Mushrooms and Peppers à la
Grecque (p. 192)
with 1 oz. cheese and
1 oz. sliced meat, ham, or
chicken
Milk, tea, or coffee

MID-AFTERNOON SNACK
(Your choice, p. 152)

DINNER
Chicken with Broccoli (p. 176)
Rice (p. 194)
Carrots (p. 188)
Perfect-Day Dessert
(check eating record):
Choice of dessert (p. 198)
or
Fruit and cheese
Beverage

(RECOMMENDED   ACTUAL
  SERVINGS)

Milk group   (2)__   __

Meat group   (2)__   __

AC group
  Grains   (4)__
  Fruits   (2)__   (8)__
                    (4)
  Vegs.   (2)__

DC group
  Fat   (1)__
                    (2)   __
  Other   (1)__

AC/DC Ratio (at least 8/1 or
8/2) __/__

Eight glasses of water?
yes__no__

Day_____   Date_____   Weight_____lbs.

24-hour change_____ lbs.   Total loss_____ lbs.

Metabolic Breakthrough Activity Program

Activity Goal_____

ACTIVITY RECORD

Kind of Activity	Amount	Time of Day
_____	_____	_____
_____	_____	_____
_____	_____	_____

Goal Reached_____(yes)_____(no)

Comments:

Metabolic Breakthrough Nutrition Plan

MENU

EATING RECORD

BREAKFAST
Cup of bouillon
1 oz. hard cheese
1 slice whole-wheat bread
Fruit (optional)
Milk, tea, or coffee

MID-MORNING SNACK
(Your choice, p. 152)

LUNCH
Cheese Toast (p. 205)
Your choice of assorted
raw vegetables, List I (p. 140)
Milk, tea, or coffee

MID-AFTERNOON SNACK
(Your choice, p. 152)

DINNER
Cabbage Rolls (p. 174)
Marinated Mushrooms (p. 155)
Perfect-Day Dessert
(check eating record):
Choice of dessert (p. 198)
or
Fruit
Beverage

(RECOMMENDED   ACTUAL
SERVINGS)

Milk group   (2)___   ___

Meat group   (2)___   ___

AC group
  Grains   (4)___
                          (8)___
  Fruits   (2)___
                    (4)
  Vegs.   (2)___

DC group
  Fat   (1)___
                    (2)   ___
  Other   (1)___

AC/DC Ratio (at least 8/1 or
8/2) ___/___

Eight glasses of water?
yes___no___

Day_____   Date_____   Weight_____lbs.
    24-hour change_____ lbs.   Total loss_____ lbs.

Metabolic Breakthrough Activity Program

Activity Goal_____

ACTIVITY RECORD

Kind of Activity	Amount	Time of Day
_____	_____	_____
_____	_____	_____
_____	_____	_____

Goal Reached_____(yes)_____(no)

Comments:

Metabolic Breakthrough Nutrition Plan

MENU   EATING RECORD

BREAKFAST
½ melon or grapefruit
1 slice whole-wheat bread
1 t. your favorite preserves
Milk, tea, or coffee

MID-MORNING SNACK
(Your choice, p. 152)

LUNCH
Cup of soup (p. 163)
Open-face sandwich:
Choice of spread (p. 161)
Assorted raw vegetables, List I
(p. 140)
Milk, tea, or coffee

MID-AFTERNOON SNACK
(Your choice, p. 152)

DINNER
Fish Roll-ups (p. 178)
Baked potato
with cottage cheese dressing
(p. 161)
Tossed salad
Choice of dressing (p. 158)
Perfect-Day Dessert
(check eating record):
Choice of dessert (p. 198)
or
Fruit and cheese
Beverage

(RECOMMENDED   ACTUAL
  SERVINGS)

Milk group   (2)___   ___

Meat group   (2)___   ___

AC group
  Grains   (4)___
  Fruits   (2)___   ⟩(8)___
                  (4)
  Vegs.   (2)___

DC group
  Fat   (1)___
                  ⟩(2)   ___
  Other   (1)___

AC/DC Ratio (at least 8/1 or
8/2) ___/___

Eight glasses of water?
yes___no___

Metabolic Breakthrough Activity Program

Activity Goal_____

ACTIVITY RECORD

Kind of Activity	Amount	Time of Day
_____	_____	_____
_____	_____	_____
_____	_____	_____

Goal Reached_____(yes)_____(no)

Comments:

Metabolic Breakthrough Nutrition Plan

MENU	EATING RECORD

MENU

BREAKFAST
½ or 1 whole canteloupe
½ cup cottage cheese
Milk, tea, or coffee

MID-MORNING SNACK
(Your choice, p. 152)

LUNCH
Cup of Split Pea Soup (or your
choice, p. 169)
2 oz. hard cheese
1 slice whole-wheat bread, or
crackers
Assorted raw vegetables, List I
(p. 140)

MID-AFTERNOON SNACK
(Your choice, p. 152)

DINNER
Baked Pork Chops with Caraway
Seeds (p. 172)
Tomatoes Florentine (p. 197)
Oven-Fried Potato Sticks (p. 192)
Perfect-Day Dessert
(check eating record):
Choice of dessert (p. 198)
or
Fruit
Beverage

EATING RECORD

(RECOMMENDED   ACTUAL
SERVINGS)

Milk group   (2)___   ___

Meat group (2)___   ___

AC group
  Grains   (4)___
  Fruits   (2)___ (8)___
    (4)
  Vegs.   (2)___

DC group
  Fat   (1)___
    (2) ___
  Other   (1)___

AC/DC Ratio (at least 8/1 or
8/2) ___/___

Eight glasses of water?
yes___no___

Day_____ Date_____ Weight_____ lbs.

24-hour change_____ lbs. Total loss_____ lbs.

Metabolic Breakthrough Activity Program

Activity Goal_____

ACTIVITY RECORD

Kind of Activity	Amount	Time of Day
_____	_____	_____
_____	_____	_____
_____	_____	_____

Goal Reached_____(yes)_____(no)

Comments:

Metabolic Breakthrough Nutrition Plan

MENU

BREAKFAST
2 slices whole-wheat bread
2 oz. cheese
Milk, tea, or coffee

MID-MORNING SNACK
(Your choice, p. 152)

LUNCH
Antipasto Salad (p. 153)
1 slice whole-wheat bread or
crackers
Milk, tea, or coffee

MID-AFTERNOON SNACK
(Your choice, p. 152)

DINNER
Spicy Chicken
with Lemon and Onions (p. 183)
Boiled potato
Cooked greens (p. 196)
or
Tossed salad (p. 157)
Perfect-Day Dessert
(check eating record):
Choice of dessert (p. 198)
or
Fruit
Beverage

EATING RECORD

(RECOMMENDED   ACTUAL
  SERVINGS)

Milk group (2)___   ___

Meat group (2)___   ___

AC group
  Grains   (4)___
  Fruits   (2)___ (8)___
                (4)
  Vegs.   (2)___

DC group
  Fat   (1)___
                (2) ___
  Other   (1)___

AC/DC Ratio (at least 8/1 or
8/2) ___/___

Eight glasses of water?
yes___no___

Day_____ Date_____ Weight_____lbs.

24-hour change_____ lbs. Total loss_____ lbs.

Metabolic Breakthrough Activity Program

Activity Goal_____

ACTIVITY RECORD

Kind of Activity	Amount	Time of Day
_____	_____	_____
_____	_____	_____
_____	_____	_____

Goal Reached_____(yes) _____(no)

Comments:

Metabolic Breakthrough Nutrition Plan

MENU

BREAKFAST
½ melon
½ cup cottage cheese
Milk, tea, or coffee

MID-MORNING SNACK
(Your choice, p. 152)

LUNCH
Cup of Broccoli Soup (or
your choice, p. 164)
Open-face Bean Spread sandwich
(p. 163)
with slice of cheese and sliced
tomato
Milk, tea, or coffee

MID-AFTERNOON SNACK
(Your choice, p. 152)

DINNER
Spaghetti
with Garlic and Clam Sauce
(p. 182)
Large green salad, favorite
dressing (p. 158)
Perfect-Day Dessert
(check eating record):
Choice of dessert (p. 198)
or
Fruit
Beverage

EATING RECORD

(RECOMMENDED   ACTUAL
SERVINGS)

Milk group (2)__   __

Meat group (2)__   __

AC group
  Grains   (4)__
  Fruits   (2)__ (8)__
               (4)
  Vegs.   (2)__

DC group
  Fat   (1)__
             (2) __
  Other   (1)__

AC/DC Ratio (at least 8/1 or
8/2) __/__

Eight glasses of water?
yes__no__

Day_____   Date_____   Weight_____lbs.

24-hour change_____ lbs.   Total loss_____ lbs.

Metabolic Breakthrough Activity Program

Activity Goal_____

ACTIVITY RECORD

Kind of Activity	Amount	Time of Day
_____	_____	_____
_____	_____	_____
_____	_____	_____

Goal Reached_____(yes)_____(no)

Comments:

Metabolic Breakthrough Nutrition Plan

MENU	EATING RECORD

BREAKFAST
Sliced orange
2 slices French Toast (p. 205)
2 t. your favorite syrup
Milk, tea, or coffee

MID-MORNING SNACK
(Your choice, p. 152)

LUNCH
Pepper and Tomato Salad
(p. 156)
with favorite dressing (p. 158)
3 oz. sliced chicken or turkey
Milk, tea, or coffee

MID-AFTERNOON SNACK
(Your choice, p. 152)

DINNER
Crab Quiche with Crumb
Topping (p. 176)
Cauliflower with Mushrooms
(p. 189)
Green Beans Almondine (p. 191)
Perfect-Day Dessert
(check eating record):
Choice of dessert (p. 198)
or
Fruit
Beverage

EATING RECORD

	(RECOMMENDED SERVINGS)	ACTUAL
Milk group	(2)__	__
Meat group	(2)__	__
AC group		
Grains	(4)__	
Fruits	(2)__	(8)__
	(4)	
Vegs.	(2)__	
DC group		
Fat	(1)__	
	(2)	__
Other	(1)__	

AC/DC Ratio (at least 8/1 or
8/2) __/__

Eight glasses of water?
yes__no__

DIRECTIONS

WEEK 3

I. Enter day number, date, weight, 24-hour change, and total weight lost since the start of the program.

II. Daily Metabolic Breakthrough Activity Program

   A. *Regular Program* 30 minutes of activity (whole-body movement), *brisk* pace, done at any convenient time, in any combination of 5-, 10-, 15-, or a single 30-minute period.
   B. *Super Booster Program* 30 minutes of activity (whole-body movement), done in either two 15-minute walks after meals (moderate pace), one 15-minute walk after a meal and a 15-minute *brisk* walk before dinner, or a single *brisk* 30-minute walk before dinner.
   C. *Advanced Program* 45 minutes of brisk activity (whole-body movement) in any combination of 5-, 10-, 15-, or 30-minute segments, or a single 45-minute segment. *You have reached the first goal of the 28-Day Metabolic Breakthrough Activity Program: each day you burn enough calories to keep yourself from regaining up to 50 pounds of fat once you reach your desired weight.*

III. Daily Metabolic Breakthrough Nutrition Plan

   A. Follow the menus exactly or make appropriate substitutions, filling in the food record in the lower right portion of each page.
   B. This week's menu features the following recipes from the Metabolic Breakthrough Nutrition Plan:
      1. Lemon-Baked Chicken (American) p. 179.
      2. Poached Eggs Italian Style p. 180.
      3. Baked Salmon in Foil (New England) p. 173.
      4. Veal Loaf (American) p. 187.
      5. Spicy Oven-Fried Chicken (Southern) p. 184.
      6. Artichoke Casserole (American) p. 171.
      7. Fillet of Lemon Sole w/Almonds (New England) p. 177.

Day_____ Date_____ Weight_____lbs.

24-hour change_____ lbs. Total loss_____ lbs.

Metabolic Breakthrough Activity Program

Activity Goal_____

ACTIVITY RECORD

Kind of Activity	Amount	Time of Day
_____	_____	_____
_____	_____	_____
_____	_____	_____

Goal Reached_____(yes)_____(no)

Comments:

Metabolic Breakthrough Nutrition Plan

MENU   EATING RECORD

BREAKFAST
Choice of fruit
2 slices whole-wheat bread
2 oz. cheese
Milk, tea, or coffee

MID-MORNING SNACK
(Your choice, p. 152)

LUNCH
Tuna-Salad sandwich (p. 157)
with bean sprouts or lettuce
and tomato
Milk, tea, or coffee

MID-AFTERNOON SNACK
(Your choice, p. 152)

DINNER
Lemon-Baked Chicken (p. 179)
Spinach and Broccoli Casserole
(p. 196)
Acorn Squash (p. 187)
Perfect-Day Dessert
(check eating record):
Choice of dessert (p. 198)
or
Fruit
Beverage

(RECOMMENDED   ACTUAL
SERVINGS)

Milk group   (2)—   —

Meat group (2)—   —

AC group
  Grains   (4)—
  Fruits   (2)—   (8)—
                 (4)
  Vegs.   (2)—

DC group
  Fat   (1)—
                 (2) —
  Other   (1)—

AC/DC Ratio (at least 8/1 or
8/2) __/__

Eight glasses of water?
yes__no__

Day_____ Date_____ Weight_____lbs.

24-hour change_____ lbs. Total loss_____ lbs.

Metabolic Breakthrough Activity Program

Activity Goal_____

ACTIVITY RECORD

Kind of Activity	Amount	Time of Day
_____	_____	_____
_____	_____	_____
_____	_____	_____

Goal Reached_____(yes) _____(no)

Comments:

Metabolic Breakthrough Nutrition Plan

MENU	EATING RECORD

BREAKFAST
Choice of fruit
Choice of cereal (pp. 148–49)
½ cup low-fat milk
Milk, tea, or coffee

MID-MORNING SNACK
(Your choice, p. 152)

LUNCH
Cup of Vichyssoise (p. 170)
or
Your choice of soup (p. 163)
Open-face sandwich, choice of
spread (p. 161)
Assorted raw vegetables, List I
(p. 140)
Milk, tea, or coffee

MID-AFTERNOON SNACK
(Your choice, p. 152)

DINNER
Poached Eggs Italian Style
(p. 180)
on two slices toast
Tossed salad, choice of dressing
(p. 158)
Perfect-Day Dessert
(check eating record):
Choice of dessert (p. 198)
or
Fruit and cheese
Beverage

(RECOMMENDED   ACTUAL
SERVINGS)

Milk group   (2)__   __

Meat group   (2)__   __

AC group
  Grains   (4)__
  Fruits   (2)__   (8)__
                (4)
  Vegs.   (2)__

DC group
  Fat   (1)__
             (2)   __
  Other   (1)__

AC/DC Ratio (at least 8/1 or
8/2) __/__

Eight glasses of water?
yes__no__

Day_____ Date_____ Weight_____lbs.

24-hour change_____ lbs. Total loss_____ lbs.

Metabolic Breakthrough Activity Program

Activity Goal_____

ACTIVITY RECORD

Kind of Activity	Amount	Time of Day
_____	_____	_____
_____	_____	_____
_____	_____	_____

Goal Reached_____(yes)_____(no)

Comments:

Metabolic Breakthrough Nutrition Plan

MENU   **EATING RECORD**

BREAKFAST
½ melon
½ cup cottage cheese
Milk, tea, or coffee

MID-MORNING SNACK
(Your choice, p. 152)

LUNCH
Ham and Cheese Sandwich
(p. 151)
with sliced tomato and tarragon
Mayonnaise Dressing (p. 158)
Assorted raw vegetables, List I
(p. 140)
Milk, tea, or coffee

MID-AFTERNOON SNACK
(Your choice, p. 152)

DINNER
Baked Salmon in Foil (p. 173)
with bouillon or rémoulade
Peas and Baby Onions (p. 193)
Choice of salad (p. 153)
and favorite dressing (p. 158)
Perfect-Day Dessert
(check eating record):
Choice of dessert (p. 198)
or
Fruit
Beverage

(RECOMMENDED   ACTUAL
SERVINGS)

Milk group (2)___ ___

Meat group (2)___ ___

AC group
Grains (4)___
Fruits (2)___ (8)___
(4)
Vegs. (2)___

DC group
Fat (1)___
(2) ___
Other (1)___

AC/DC Ratio (at least 8/1 or
8/2) ___/___

Eight glasses of water?
yes___no___

Day_____ Date_____ Weight_____lbs.

24-hour change_____ lbs. Total loss_____ lbs.

Metabolic Breakthrough Activity Program

Activity Goal_____

Kind of Activity	Amount	Time of Day
_____	_____	_____
_____	_____	_____
_____	_____	_____

Goal Reached_____(yes)_____(no)

Comments:

_____

Metabolic Breakthrough Nutrition Plan

MENU   EATING RECORD

MENU	EATING RECORD	
BREAKFAST	(RECOMMENDED	ACTUAL
Choice of fruit	SERVINGS)	
2 slices whole-wheat bread	Milk group (2)__	__
1 T. peanut butter	Meat group (2)__	__
(or favorite spread, p. 161)	AC group	
Milk, tea, or coffee	Grains (4)__	
MID-MORNING SNACK	Fruits (2)__ ╲(8)__	
(Your choice, p. 152)	(4)	
LUNCH	Vegs. (2)__	
Choice of soup (p. 163)	DC group	
1 slice whole-wheat bread	Fat (1)__	
2 oz. favorite cheese	(2) __	
MID-AFTERNOON SNACK	Other (1)__	
(Your choice, p. 152)		
DINNER	AC/DC Ratio (at least 8/1 or	
Veal Loaf (p. 187)	8/2) __/__	
Tossed salad (p. 157)	Eight glasses of water?	
Cooked Carrots with Herbs	yes__no__	
(p. 191)		
Perfect-Day Dessert		
(check eating record):		
Choice of dessert (p. 198)		
or		
Fruit		
Beverage		

Day_____ Date_____ Weight_____lbs.

24-hour change_____ lbs.　　　Total loss_____ lbs.

Metabolic Breakthrough Activity Program

Activity Goal_____

ACTIVITY RECORD

Kind of Activity	Amount	Time of Day
_____	_____	_____
_____	_____	_____
_____	_____	_____

Goal Reached_____(yes)_____(no)

Comments:

Metabolic Breakthrough Nutrition Plan

MENU　　　　　　　　　　　　**EATING RECORD**

BREAKFAST
½ grapefruit
1 slice whole-wheat bread
1 egg, hard- or soft-boiled, or
poached
Milk, tea, or coffee

MID-MORNING SNACK
(Your choice, p. 152)

LUNCH
Watercress Soup (p. 170)
(or your choice of soup, p. 163)
Open-face sandwich, choice of
spread (p. 161)
Assorted raw vegetables, List I
(p. 140)
Milk, tea, or coffee

MID-AFTERNOON SNACK
(Your choice, p. 152)

DINNER
Spicy Oven-Fried Chicken (p. 184)
Macaroni Salad (p. 155)
Carrot Soufflé (p. 188)
Perfect-Day Dessert
(check eating record):
Choice of dessert (p. 198)
or
Fruit and cheese
Beverage

(RECOMMENDED　　　　ACTUAL
SERVINGS)

Milk group　(2)__　　　　__

Meat group　(2)__　　　　__

AC group
　Grains　(4)__
　Fruits　(2)__　　(8)__
　　　　　　　　(4)
　Vegs.　(2)__

DC group
　Fat　(1)__
　　　　　　(2)　__
　Other　(1)__

AC/DC Ratio (at least 8/1 or
8/2) __/__

Eight glasses of water?
yes__no__

Day_____ Date_____ Weight_____lbs.

24-hour change_____ lbs. Total loss_____ lbs.

Metabolic Breakthrough Activity Program

Activity Goal_____

ACTIVITY RECORD

Kind of Activity	Amount	Time of Day
_____	_____	_____
_____	_____	_____
_____	_____	_____

Goal Reached_____(yes)_____(no)

Comments:

Metabolic Breakthrough Nutrition Plan

MENU

BREAKFAST
2 slices whole-wheat bread
2 oz. cheese
Milk, tea, or coffee

MID-MORNING SNACK
(Your choice, p. 152)

LUNCH
Tomato stuffed with tuna, or
your favorite spread (p. 161)
Romaine, sliced cucumber, and
other assorted raw vegetables
Milk, tea, or coffee

SNACK
(Your choice, p. 152)

DINNER
Artichoke Casserole (p. 171)
Brown rice (p. 194)
Tossed salad, with
choice of dressing (p. 157)
Perfect-Day Dessert
(check eating record):
Choice of dessert (p. 198)
or
Fruit
Beverage

EATING RECORD

(RECOMMENDED   ACTUAL
SERVINGS)

Milk group   (2)___   ___

Meat group   (2)___   ___

AC group
  Grains   (4)___
  Fruits   (2)___   (8)___
                  (4)
  Vegs.   (2)___

DC group
  Fat   (1)___
                  (2)   ___
  Other   (1)___

AC/DC Ratio (at least 8/1 or
8/2) ___/___

Eight glasses of water?
yes___no___

Day_____   Date_____   Weight_____lbs.

24-hour change_____ lbs.   Total loss_____ lbs.

Metabolic Breakthrough Activity Program

Activity Goal_____

ACTIVITY RECORD

Kind of Activity	Amount	Time of Day
_____	_____	_____
_____	_____	_____
_____	_____	_____

Goal Reached_____ (yes) _____ (no)

Comments:

Metabolic Breakthrough Nutrition Plan

MENU	EATING RECORD

MENU

BREAKFAST
Choice of fruit
Choice of cereal (pp. 148–49)
½ cup of low-fat milk
Milk, tea, or coffee

MID-MORNING SNACK
(Your choice, p. 152)

LUNCH
Stuffed Zucchini Salad (p. 157)
Tarragon Vinegar Dressing
(p. 160)
Milk, tea, or coffee

MID-AFTERNOON SNACK
(Your choice, p. 152)

DINNER
Fillet of Lemon Sole with
Almonds (p. 177)
Baked potato
with cottage cheese dressing
(p. 161)
Assorted raw vegetables, List I
(p. 140)
Perfect-Day Dessert
(check eating record):
Choice of dessert
or
Fruit and cheese
Beverage

EATING RECORD

(RECOMMENDED   ACTUAL
SERVINGS)

Milk group (2)__   __

Meat group (2)__   __

AC group
  Grains   (4)__
  Fruits   (2)__ ＞(8)__
            (4)
  Vegs.   (2)__

DC group
  Fat   (1)__
           (2)   __
  Other   (1)__

AC/DC Ratio (at least 8/1 or
8/2) __/__

Eight glasses of water?
yes__no__

DIRECTIONS

WEEK 4

I. Enter day number, date, weight, 24-hour change, and total weight lost since the start of the program.

II. Daily Metabolic Breakthrough Activity Program

> *In this week everyone will have reached the first goal of the 28-Day Metabolic Breakthrough Activity Program: each day you will be burning enough calories to keep yourself from regaining up to 50 pounds of fat once you have reached your desired weight.*

    A. *Regular Program* 45 minutes of activity (whole-body movement), *brisk* pace, done at any convenient time, in any combination of 5-, 10-, 15-, 30-, or a single 45-minute period.

    B. *Super Booster Program* 45 minutes of activity (whole-body movement), done in 15-minute walks at a moderate pace after meals, or in combinations of 15- or 30-minute walks at a *brisk* pace before dinner, or a single *brisk* 45-minute walk before dinner.

    C. *Advanced Program* 45 minutes of *brisk* activity (whole-body movement) in any combination of 5-, 10-, 15-, or 30-minute segments, or a single 45-minute segment.

III. Daily Metabolic Breakthrough Nutrition Plan

    A. Follow the menus exactly or make appropriate substitutions, filling in the food record in the lower right portion of each page.

    B. This week's menu features the following recipes from the Metabolic Breakthrough Nutrition Plan:
       1. Rice and Beans (Vegetarian) p. 181.
       2. Almond Chicken (Oriental) p. 171.
       3. Baked Rainbow Trout (American) p. 174.
       4. Veal and Garbanzos (East Indian) p. 186.
       5. Crab with Vermicelli (Italian) p. 177.
       6. Cauliflower Italian Style (Vegetarian) p. 175.
       7. Tandoori Chicken (East Indian) p. 185.

Day_____. Date_____ Weight_____lbs.

24-hour change_____ lbs. Total loss_____ lbs.

Metabolic Breakthrough Activity Program

Activity Goal_____

ACTIVITY RECORD

Kind of Activity	Amount	Time of Day
_____	_____	_____
_____	_____	_____
_____	_____	_____

Goal Reached_____(yes)_____(no)

Comments:

Metabolic Breakthrough Nutrition Plan

MENU

EATING RECORD

BREAKFAST
1 slice whole-wheat bread
1 egg, hard- or soft-boiled, or
poached
Milk, tea, or coffee

MID-MORNING SNACK
(Your choice, p. 152)

LUNCH
Creative Fruit Salad (p. 154)
½ cup cottage cheese
Milk, tea, or coffee

MID-AFTERNOON SNACK
(Your choice, p. 152)

DINNER
Rice and Beans (p. 181)
2 oz. grated cheese
Cooked greens (p. 196)
or
Tossed salad (p. 157)
Choice of dressing (p. 158)
Perfect-Day Dessert
(check eating record):
Choice of dessert
or
Fruit
Beverage

(RECOMMENDED   ACTUAL
SERVINGS)

Milk group (2)__   __

Meat group (2)__   __

AC group
  Grains (4)__
  Fruits (2)__ (8)__
           (4)
  Vegs. (2)__

DC group
  Fat (1)__
        (2)   __
  Other (1)__

AC/DC Ratio (at least 8/1 or
8/2) __/__

Eight glasses of water?
yes__no__

Day_____ Date_____ Weight_____lbs.

24-hour change_____ lbs.   Total loss_____ lbs.

Metabolic Breakthrough Activity Program

Activity Goal_____

Kind of Activity	Amount	Time of Day
_____	_____	_____
_____	_____	_____
_____	_____	_____

Goal Reached_____(yes)_____(no)

Comments:

Metabolic Breakthrough Nutrition Plan

MENU	EATING RECORD

BREAKFAST
½ grapefruit or melon
Choice of cereal (pp. 148–49)
½ cup low-fat milk
Milk, tea, or coffee

MID-MORNING SNACK
(Your choice, p. 152)

LUNCH
Creative Chef Salad (p. 154)
Choice of dressing (p. 158)
Milk, tea, or coffee

MID-AFTERNOON SNACK
(Your choice, p. 152)

DINNER
Almond Chicken (p. 171)
Brown rice (p. 194)
Broccoli (p. 196)
Perfect-Day Dessert
(check eating record):
Choice of dessert (p. 198)
or
Fruit and cheese
Beverage

(RECOMMENDED   ACTUAL
SERVINGS)

Milk group   (2)___   ___

Meat group   (2)___   ___

AC group
Grains   (4)___
Fruits   (2)___   (8)___
(4)
Vegs.   (2)___

DC group
Fat   (1)___
(2)   ___
Other   (1)___

AC/DC Ratio (at least 8/1 or
8/2) ___/___

Eight glasses of water?
yes___no___

Day_____   Date_____   Weight_____lbs.

24-hour change_____ lbs.   Total loss_____ lbs.

Metabolic Breakthrough Activity Program

Activity Goal_____

ACTIVITY RECORD

Kind of Activity	Amount	Time of Day
_____	_____	_____
_____	_____	_____
_____	_____	_____

Goal Reached_____(yes)_____(no)

Comments:

Metabolic Breakthrough Nutrition Plan

MENU   EATING RECORD

BREAKFAST
Choice of fruit
½ cup cottage cheese
Milk, tea, or coffee

MID-MORNING SNACK
(Your choice, p. 152)

LUNCH
Sandwich, with choice of spread
(p. 161)
Assorted raw vegetables, List I
(p. 140)
Milk, tea, or coffee

MID-AFTERNOON SNACK
(Your choice, p. 152)

DINNER
Baked or Broiled Whole
Rainbow Trout (p. 174)
Baked Tomato (p. 195)
Green Beans with Mushrooms
(p. 191)
Perfect-Day Dessert
(check eating record):
Choice of dessert (p. 198)
or
Fruit
Beverage

(RECOMMENDED   ACTUAL
SERVINGS)

Milk group (2)___   ___

Meat group (2)___   ___

AC group
  Grains   (4)___
  Fruits   (2)___ (8)___
             (4)
  Vegs.   (2)___

DC group
  Fat   (1)___
            (2) ___
  Other   (1)___

AC/DC Ratio (at least 8/1 or
8/2) ___/___

Eight glasses of water?
yes___no___

131

Day_____   Date_____   Weight_____lbs.

24-hour change_____ lbs.   Total loss_____ lbs.

Metabolic Breakthrough Activity Program

Activity Goal_____

ACTIVITY RECORD

Kind of Activity   Amount   Time of Day

_____   _____   _____
_____   _____   _____
_____   _____   _____

Goal Reached_____(yes)_____(no)

Comments:

Metabolic Breakthrough Nutrition Plan

MENU	EATING RECORD

BREAKFAST
Pancakes (p. 205)
1 T. your favorite syrup
Milk, tea, or coffee

MID-MORNING SNACK
(Your choice, p. 152)

LUNCH
Antipasto (p. 153)
1 slice whole-wheat bread, or
crackers
Milk, tea, or coffee

MID-AFTERNOON SNACK
(Your choice, p. 152)

DINNER
Veal and Garbanzos (p. 186)
Brown rice (p. 194)
Cooked greens (p. 196)
or
Tossed salad (p. 157)
with choice of dressing (p. 158)
Perfect-Day Dessert
(check eating record):
Choice of dessert (p. 198)
or
Fruit
Beverage

(RECOMMENDED   ACTUAL
SERVINGS)

Milk group   (2)___   ___

Meat group   (2)___   ___

AC group
  Grains   (4)___
  Fruits   (2)___   (8)___
                     (4)
  Vegs.   (2)___

DC group
  Fat   (1)___
                     (2)   ___
  Other   (1)___

AC/DC Ratio (at least 8/1 or
8/2) ___/___

Eight glasses of water?
yes___no___

Day_____ Date_____ Weight_____lbs.

24-hour change_____ lbs. Total loss_____ lbs.

Metabolic Breakthrough Activity Program

Activity Goal_____

ACTIVITY RECORD

Kind of Activity	Amount	Time of Day
_____	_____	_____
_____	_____	_____
_____	_____	_____

Goal Reached_____(yes)_____(no)

Comments:

Metabolic Breakthrough Nutrition Plan

MENU	EATING RECORD

MENU

BREAKFAST
½ grapefruit
1 slice whole-wheat bread
1 egg, hard- or soft-boiled, or
poached
Milk, tea, or coffee

MID-MORNING SNACK
(Your choice, p. 152)

LUNCH
Choice of soup (p. 163)
1 oz. cheese
1 slice whole-wheat bread
Assorted raw vegetables, List I
(p. 140)
Milk, tea, or coffee

MID-AFTERNOON SNACK
(Your choice, p. 152)

DINNER
Crab with Vermicelli (p. 177)
Sliced Tomatoes and Cucumbers
(p. 156)
Tarragon Vinegar Dressing
(p. 160)
Perfect-Day Dessert
(check eating record):
Choice of dessert (p. 198)
or
Fruit
Beverage

EATING RECORD

(RECOMMENDED   ACTUAL
SERVINGS)

Milk group   (2)___   ___

Meat group (2)___   ___

AC group
Grains   (4)___
Fruits   (2)___   (8)___
              (4)
Vegs.   (2)___

DC group
Fat   (1)___
              (2)   ___
Other   (1)___

AC/DC Ratio (at least 8/1 or
8/2) ___/___

Eight glasses of water?
yes___no___

Day_____ Date_____ Weight_____lbs.

24-hour change_____ lbs. Total loss_____ lbs.

Metabolic Breakthrough Activity Program

Activity Goal_____

ACTIVITY RECORD

Kind of Activity	Amount	Time of Day
_____	_____	_____
_____	_____	_____
_____	_____	_____

Goal Reached_____(yes)_____(no)

Comments:

Metabolic Breakthrough Nutrition Plan

MENU	EATING RECORD

BREAKFAST
½ grapefruit
Choice of cereal (pp. 148–49)
½ cup low-fat milk
Milk, tea, or coffee

MID-MORNING SNACK
(Your choice, p. 152)

LUNCH
Broiled open-face sandwich:
Bean Spread (p. 163) with
1 oz. cheddar cheese
sliced tomato and herbs
Assorted raw vegetables, List I
(p. 140)
Milk, tea, or coffee

MID-AFTERNOON SNACK
(Your choice, p. 152)

DINNER
Cauliflower Italian Style (p. 175)
Whole-grain rice (p. 194)
Perfect-Day Dessert
(check eating record):
Choice of dessert (p. 198)
or
Fruit
Beverage

EATING RECORD

(RECOMMENDED   ACTUAL
SERVINGS)

Milk group   (2)___   ___
Meat group (2)___   ___
AC group
  Grains   (4)___
  Fruits   (2)___ (8)___
                      (4)
  Vegs.   (2)___
DC group
  Fat   (1)___
                      (2)   ___
  Other   (1)___

AC/DC Ratio (at least 8/1 or
8/2) ___/___
Eight glasses of water?
yes___no___

Day_____   Date_____   Weight_____lbs.

24-hour change_____ lbs.   Total loss_____ lbs.

Metabolic Breakthrough Activity Program

Activity Goal_____

ACTIVITY RECORD

Kind of Activity	Amount	Time of Day
_____	_____	_____
_____	_____	_____
_____	_____	_____

Goal Reached_____(yes)_____(no)

Comments:

Metabolic Breakthrough Nutrition Plan

MENU

BREAKFAST
Choice of fruit
2 slices whole-wheat bread
2 oz. cheese
Milk, tea, or coffee

MID-MORNING SNACK
(Your choice, p. 152)

LUNCH
Egg-Salad sandwich (p. 155)
Assorted raw vegetables, List I
(p. 140)
Milk, tea, or coffee

MID-AFTERNOON SNACK
(Your choice, p. 152)

DINNER
Tandoori Chicken (p. 185)
Rice and Spinach (p. 195)
Tossed salad (p. 157)
Choice of dressing (p. 158)
Perfect-Day Dessert
(check eating record):
Choice of dessert (p. 198)
or
Fruit
Beverage

EATING RECORD

(RECOMMENDED SERVINGS)		ACTUAL
Milk group	(2)__	__
Meat group	(2)__	__
AC group		
Grains	(4)__	
Fruits	(2)__	(8)__
	(4)	
Vegs.	(2)__	
DC group		
Fat	(1)__	
	(2)	__
Other	(1)__	

AC/DC Ratio (at least 8/1 or 8/2) __/__

Eight glasses of water?
yes__no__

Food Exchange and Quick Calorie Counter Lists

Many different foods are arranged in lists below so that you can make substitutions in your 28-Day Nutrition Plan from among foods that are similar in food values. The lists are called "Exchange Lists" because, when you make a substitution in your Nutrition Plan, you should "exchange" foods that are generally similar in nutrient value. For example, if my daily menu breakfast calls for cereal and milk, you can exchange cereal for bread, or milk for cheese, because they come from the same food list (or "group" of foods).

The lists contain useful "quick" calorie counts of foods in the various categories, but YOU DO NOT COUNT CALORIES WHEN YOU FOLLOW THIS NUTRITION PLAN. The calories are supplied for other reasons.

When you follow the guidelines for the Metabolic Breakthrough Nutrition Plan, eating the number of servings that are recommended in each food category, it isn't necessary to count calories to achieve a weight loss of between 1 and 3 pounds per week. I have included these calorie counts because so many people are interested in being able to obtain a quick estimate of their food intake each day. A knowledge of these general values does away with having to search through those more exhaustive calorie counters. In the final analysis, the very detailed calorie books are not much more accurate than these general values because there is great variability in the calories contained in any given serving of food—even from orange to orange! Not to mention from one piece of apple pie to the next. Your calorie books just give you the average obtained from testing many samples.

And even though you don't count calories when you follow this nutrition plan, a quick look at the relative caloric value of foods in each category can be very helpful to anyone who has no previous knowledge of the energy content of different foods. This knowledge will help you make wise choices when eating out or when choosing that second serving of foods in the DC category.

Of course, if you want to speed your weight loss, you should always choose the foods within each group that have the fewest calories. It can add up to another half-pound a week of weight loss if you do it consistently.

The lists include the following:

The Milk List: Foods high in calcium. Have two servings a day.

The Meat List: Divided into low-fat, medium-fat, and high-fat meat, fowl, and fish. Cheese can also count as *either* a meat group *or* a milk group food. Meats are high in complete protein, B vitamins, and minerals. Three ounces is considered a serving of meat in spite of the great variability in calories due to fat content. Of course, to speed your weight loss, it's advisable to stick with low- and medium-fat varieties. Women should have 6 oz. and men 9 oz. per day to satisfy protein needs.

There are three lists for the AC group of foods. These are your high-fiber foods: fruits, vegetables, and breads and cereals. Some vegetables appear in Vegetable List I. These are the low-calorie vegetables, generally high in vitamin A. Vegetable List II is included with the cereals and grains because these vegetables are more similar to these cereal and grain foods in nutrient values. The legumes in this list also contain a moderate amount of protein.

The AC Group Vegetable List I: Complex-carbohydrate, low-calorie vegetables, high in vitamin A and fiber.

The AC Group Fruit List: Low-calorie fruits, generally high in vitamin C and fiber.

The AC Group Bread, Cereal, and Vegetable List II: High in complex carbohydrates, B vitamins, and a broad array of minerals. Whole grains and legumes will be high in fiber and have moderate protein value.

You should have a total of eight servings of foods from the AC group per day. Nutritionists suggest a minimum of two fruits (one citrus), two vegetables, and four selections from the Bread, Cereal, and Vegetable List II. This suggestion is indicated on the Eating Record side of your daily Nutrition Plan. A wide variety of foods from the AC group helps assure adequate nutrition and, as long as you have a minimum of eight servings a day, it is not of primary importance that you always have exactly two fruits, two vegetables, and four grains.

The DC group of foods includes fats and some miscellaneous candy, snack, and dessert foods. Use your first DC allowance for butter, margarine, or oil, as spread or in cooking. Add a second allowance only after you have had eight servings of foods from the AC lists. This will give you the correct 8/2 AC/DC ratio.

Milk Exchange List

170 CALORIES

1 c. whole milk
½ c. evaporated milk

125 CALORIES

1 c. 2% fat milk
1 c. partially skim yogurt

100 CALORIES

1 c. 1% (low-fat) milk
1 oz. cheddar-type cheeses

80 CALORIES

1 c. skim milk, buttermilk, or skim
    yogurt
⅓ c. ice milk or creamed cottage
    cheese

75 CALORIES

1 oz. cheese: mozzarella, ricotta,
    farmer's cheese, Neufchatel
3 T. Parmesan cheese

55 CALORIES

¼ c. cottage cheese, dry and 1%
    butterfat
1 oz. cheese with less than 5%
    butterfat

Meat Exchange List

LEAN

The leanest cuts have approximately 55 calories in the quantities listed.

1 oz. beef: baby beef (very lean), chipped beef, chuck, flank steak, tenderloin, plate ribs, plate skirt steak, round (bottom, top), all cuts rump, spare ribs, tripe
1 oz. lamb: leg, rib, sirloin, loin (roast and chops), shank, shoulder
1 oz. pork: leg (whole rump, center shank), ham, smoked (center slices)
1 oz. veal: leg, loin, rib, shank, shoulder, cutlets
1 oz. poultry: chicken, turkey, Cornish hen, guinea hen, pheasant (meat without skin)
1 oz. fresh or frozen fish: any kind
¼ c. canned fish: salmon, tuna, mackerel, crab, lobster
5 (or 1 oz.): clams, oysters, scallops, shrimp
3 sardines, drained
1 oz. any cheese containing less than 5% butterfat
¼ c. cottage cheese, dry and 1% butterfat
¼ c. legumes: any dried beans or peas

MEDIUM FAT

The following have about 75 calories in the amounts indicated.

1 oz. beef: ground (15% fat), corned beef (canned), rib eye, round (ground commercial)
1 oz. pork: loin (all cuts tenderloin), shoulder arm (picnic), shoulder blade, Boston butt, Canadian bacon, boiled ham
1 oz.: liver, heart, kidney, sweetbreads
¼ c. creamed cottage cheese
1 oz. cheese: mozzarella, ricotta, farmer's cheese, Neufchatel
3 T. Parmesan cheese
1 egg

HIGH FAT

The following have about 100 calories in the amounts listed.

1 oz. beef: brisket, corned beef (brisket), ground beef (more than 20% fat), hamburger (commercial), chuck (ground commercial), roasts (rib), steaks (club and rib)
1 oz. lamb: breast
1 oz. pork: spare ribs, loin (back ribs), pork (ground), country-style ham, deviled ham
1 oz. veal: breast
1 oz. poultry: capon, duck (domestic), goose
1 oz. cheese: cheddar types
1 slice cold cuts
1 small frankfurter
1 T. peanut butter

THE AC LISTS

Information is approximate. Total fiber in grams per serving is listed for all foods in these lists when available.* When that information is not available, the fiber content column is marked "NA." Because fiber is not digestible, the actual number of calories available to the body is less for foods with higher fiber contents.

Vegetable Exchange List I

Vegetables below have approximately 25 calories per half cup. Fiber is listed in grams per half cup.

VEGETABLE	FIBER	VEGETABLE	FIBER
Asparagus	1.7	Mushrooms	5.0
Bean sprouts	1.6	Okra	1.6
Beets	2.5	Onions	1.5
Broccoli	1.1	Rhubarb	2.9
Brussels sprouts	2.0	Rutabaga	3.2
Cabbage	1.5	Sauerkraut	2.0
Carrots	3.4	Spinach	1.8
Cauliflower	.9	String beans	1.2
Celery	1.8	Summer squash	2.2
Cucumbers	1.4	Tomatoes	1.4
Eggplant	2.0	Tomato juice	NA
Green pepper	1.2	Turnips	2.2
Greens: beet, chards, collards, dandelion, kale, mustard, turnip	2.0	Vegetable juice cocktail	NA
		Wax beans	2.1
		Zucchini	3.0

*Sources include J. Brody, 1981, *Jane Brody's Nutrition Book*, New York, W. W. Norton; D. A. T. Southgate, 1977, The definition and analysis of dietary fiber, *Nutrition Review* 35:31; *Composition of Foods: Fruits and Fruit Juices*, Agriculture Handbook No. 8-9, United States Department of Agriculture, Human Nutrition Information Service, 1982; *Composition of Foods: Breakfast Cereals*, Agriculture Handbook No. 8-8, United States Department of Agriculture, Human Nutrition Information Service, 1982; A. Eyton, 1982, *F-plan diet*, New York, Crown Publishers.

There are several different ways to determine the fiber content of food, each of which leads to values different from the others. At present, no single method is considered "best." Values listed are sometimes the average of two sources.

The following have negligible calories and can be eaten in unlimited quantities. Fiber is listed in grams per half cup.

VEGETABLE	FIBER	VEGETABLE	FIBER
Chicory	NA	Lettuce	.4
Chinese cabbage	1.5	Parsley	1.2
Endive	.6	Radishes	.5
Escarole	NA	Watercress	1.0

Fruit Exchange List

Raw or unsweetened fruits will have approximately 40 calories in the quantities listed below. Fruits canned in syrup will have about twice the calories.

FRUIT	AMOUNT	FIBER (grams)
Apple	1 small	1.5
Applesauce (unsweetened)	½ cup	1.7
Apricots, fresh	2 medium	1.6
Apricots, dried	4 halves	3.4
Banana	½ small	1.5
Blackberries	½ cup	3.8
Blueberries	½ cup	NA
Cantaloupe	¼ small	1.0
Cherries	10 large	1.2
Cider	⅓ cup	NA
Cranberries, no sugar	½ cup	4.0
Dates	2	2.4
Figs, fresh	1	2.0
Grapefruit	½	2.6
Grapes	12	.6
Honeydew melon	⅛ medium	1.5
Juices		
Apple	⅓ cup	NA
Grapefruit	½ cup	NA
Grape	¼ cup	NA
Orange	¼ cup	NA
Pineapple	⅓ cup	NA
Prune	¼ cup	NA
Mango	½ small	NA
Nectarine	1 small	NA
Orange	1 small	1.2

FRUIT	AMOUNT	FIBER (grams)
Papaya	¾ cup	1.8
Peach	1 medium	1.3
Pear	1 small	2.8
Persimmon, native	1 medium	NA
Pineapple	½ cup	1.5
Plums	2 medium	2.0
Prunes	2 medium	1.3
Raisins	2 T.	2.0
Raspberries	½ cup	4.6
Strawberries	¾ cup	3.9
Tangerine	1 medium	NA

Bread, Cereal, and Vegetable Exchange List II

Except as indicated, these items have about 70 calories in the quantities listed.

BREAD	AMOUNT	FIBER (grams)
White, French and Italian	1 slice	1.0
Whole wheat, rye, and whole-wheat raisin	1 slice	3.0
Pumpernickel	1 slice	2.0
Biscuit*	1	1.0
Roll*	1	1.0
Muffin*	1	2.0
Bagel, small	½	1.0
Dried bread crumbs	3 T.	NA
English muffin, small	½	1.9
Cornbread* (2" × 2" × 1")	1	3.0
Hotdog or hamburger bun	½	NA
Tortilla (6")	1	2.0
Pancake* (5" × .5")	1	NA
Popover	1	NA
Waffle* (5" × .5")	1	NA

*These items have about 115 calories in the amounts indicated.

CEREAL	AMOUNT	FIBER (grams)
Bran flakes	½ cup	3.0
Cooked cereal: grits, rice, or barley	½ cup	2.0
Cooked pasta: whole-wheat spaghetti, noodles, macaroni	½ cup	2.8
Cornmeal (dry)	2 T.	2.0
Flour, all purpose	2½ T.	.2
Flour, whole wheat	2½ T.	1.8
Popcorn (popped, no fat added)	3 cups	3.0
Puffed cereal, unfrosted	1 cup	3.0
Ready-to-eat unsweetened cereal	¾ cup	1.0
Wheat germ	¼ cup	NA

(See also the special Cereal listing, pp. 148–49.)

CRACKERS		
Arrowroot	3	NA
Croutons	1 cup	NA
Graham (2½″ sq.)	2	1.4
Matzoh (4″×6″)	½	NA
Oyster	20	NA
Pretzels (3⅛″ long × ⅛″ diam.)	25	NA
Round, butter type	5	NA
Ry-Krisp	3	2.3
Saltines	6	NA
Soda (2½″ sq.)	4	NA

VEGETABLE LIST II	AMOUNT	FIBER (grams)
Beans, peas, lentils (dried and cooked)	½ cup	4.0
Baked beans, no pork (canned)	⅔ cup	3.3
Corn	⅓ cup	2.1
Corn on the cob	1 small	2.1
Lima beans	½ cup	3.7
Parsnips	⅔ cup	3.0
Peas, green	½ cup	3.8
Potato, white	1 small	3.1
Potato, mashed	½ cup	3.7
Potatoes, French fried*	8 fries	NA
Pumpkin	¾ cup	5.3
Winter squash, acorn, butternut	½ cup	3.5
Yam or sweet potato	¼ cup	2.0
Tomato catsup	¼ cup	.8
Soup Meat or vegetable (3 serv./can)	1 serv.	NA
Cream, pea, bean (3 serv./can)	½ serv.	NA

*About 115 calories in the amount indicated.

THE DC LIST

Fats and Miscellaneous Foods

There are about 100 calories in these foods in the amounts listed below.

FOOD ITEM	AMOUNT	FIBER (grams)
Almonds	20 whole	4.8
Avocado (4″ diam.)	¼	1.4
Bacon, crisp	3 strips	NA
Brazil nuts	4 whole	5.0
Butter, oleo, mayonnaise, oil, lard	1 T.	NA
Coconut, dried	2 T.	3.4
Cream		
Light or sour	4 T.	NA
Heavy	2 T.	NA
Cream cheese	2 T.	NA
Dressings		
French, Italian	2 T.	NA
Oil & vinegar, blue cheese	1 T.	NA
Gravy	4 T.	NA
Olives	10 small	1.5
Pecans	4 lg. whole	NA
Peanuts		
Spanish	40 whole	2.2
Virginia	20 whole	2.2
Salad dressing, mayonnaise type	1 T.	NA
Salt pork	1⅕″ cube	NA

The following have about 40 calories in the amounts listed.

FOOD ITEM	AMOUNT	FIBER
Caramel	1	NA
Gum drops	10 small	NA
Hard candy	1 small	NA
Jelly beans	7	NA
Lifesavers	6	NA
Popsicles	½ twin bar	NA
Sugar, syrup, honey, jam, jelly, cocoa	1 level T.	NA

The following have about 80 calories in the amounts listed.

FOOD ITEM	AMOUNT	FIBER
Angel-food cake	1/12 cake	NA
Beer, carbonated beverages	6 oz.	NA
Gin, rum, whiskey, liqueur	1 oz.	NA
Jello	1 serving (5/pkg.)	NA
Sponge cake	1/12 cake	NA
Sherbet	1/3 cup	NA
Wine		
Red, sweet	2 oz.	NA
Light, dry	3 oz.	NA

The following have about 110 calories in the amounts listed.

FOOD ITEM	AMOUNT	FIBER
Bread stuffing	½ cup	NA
Cake doughnut, plain	1	NA
Ice cream	⅓ cup	NA
Potato or corn chips	10	NA

The following have about 175 calories in the amounts listed, except as indicated.

FOOD ITEM	AMOUNT	FIBER
Brownie	2″×2″×1″	NA
Cake: plain or chocolate with icing, cheese cake	1/12 of 9″ cake	NA
Chocolate candy bars*	1.4 oz.	NA
Pies: custard, cream, fruit	1/12 of 9″ pie (about ½ average piece)	NA

*210 calories.

CHARACTERISTICS OF HIGH- AND LOW-CALORIE FOODS

HIGH CALORIE	LOW CALORIE
Thick, oily, or greasy-crisp	Thin, watery, or dilute
Slick, smooth, or gooey	Bulky, or with lots of fiber or coarseness
Sweet or sticky	Watery-crisp instead of greasy-crisp
Compact or concentrated	
Alcoholic	

BRAND-NAME CEREALS

The list below contains the calories per serving and fiber content of various cereals. Keep a variety in the house for breakfast and for use as an occasional snack. The variety will make eating cereals more appealing.

Cereals, Dry

BRAND	QUANTITY	CALORIES	FIBER (grams)
General Mills			
Total	1 cup	110	2.0
Wheaties	1 cup	110	2.0
Kellogg's			
All-Bran	⅓ cup	70	9.0
Bran Buds	⅓ cup	70	8.0
Cracklin' Oat			
Bran	½ cup	120	4.0
40% Bran Flakes	⅔ cup	90	4.0
Most	½ cup	100	4.0
Nutri-Grain Wheat	⅔ cup	110	2.0
Raisin Bran	¾ cup	110	4.0
Nabisco			
100% Bran	½ cup	70	9.0
Spoon Size			
Shredded Wheat	⅔ cup	110	NA
Toasted Wheat			
and Raisins	(1 oz.)	100	2.0
Post			
Grape-Nuts	¼ cup	100	4.6
Grape-Nuts Flakes	⅞ cup	100	NA
Raisin Bran	½ cup	90	NA
Quaker: Corn Bran	⅔ cup	110	5.0
Ralston Purina			
Bran Chex	⅔ cup	90	5.0
Corn Chex	1 cup	110	NA
Wheat Chex	⅔ cup	100	2.0

Cereals, Cooked

Figures given are for cooked quantities.

BRAND	QUANTITY	CALORIES	FIBER (grams)
Corn Grits	¾ cup	110	.5
Cream of Wheat, instant	¾ cup	115	NA
Oats, regular	¾ cup	108	1.1
Ralston	¾ cup	100	3.2
Wheatena	¾ cup	101	NA

FOODS HIGH IN SODIUM

Anchovies and anchovy paste
Bacon
Baking powder
Baked beans with pork
Beef: corned, dried
Bouillon cubes (most brands, check labels)
Canned vegetables
Catsup in large quantities
Celery salt
Cereals and certain cereal-type foods such as All-bran and salted Ry-Krisp
Cheeses such as cheddar and processed
Cod fish, salted
Corn, popped with salt (okay plain)
Crab, canned
Crackers, soda type
Flours, self-rising
Ham
Olives
Peanuts, salted
Pickles
Potato chips
Processed luncheon meats
Pretzels
Sausage, frankfurters
Soups, canned
Tuna, canned
Wheat flakes and cereals, check labels
Worcestershire sauce

Recipes

All of the recipes that are included in this section were created by me and the other members of my family. They have all passed the "taste test" in our home, and among our friends. Many of the recipes are adaptations taken from the most famous chefs of the world in my effort to preserve the flavor I like while reducing the fat and sugar content. I think I, and my wife and children, have been successful in our attempts.

There is no secret to the process. You can do it with any recipe you like. And you can substitute your own favorite recipes thoughout your 28-Day Program. When you make substitutions, keep a record on the forms provided by the 28-Day Metabolic Breakthrough Nutrition Plan (pp. 104–35). This is your assurance that you are still implementing the plan correctly.

Here are the general rules for adapting any of your own favorite dishes.

Rules for Preparing all Recipes the Low-Calorie Way

The two main sources of extra and unnecessary calories are fats and sugar. The first time you attempt to modify your own recipes, try halving the amount of fat and reducing sugar by 25 percent. If that works, halve the fat again the next time you prepare the dish, and cut another 25 percent of the sugar.

You never need more than one tablespoon of fat for sautéing onions, peppers, celery, and garlic before combining with other ingredients. Cover the skillet, cook on medium heat or lower, and add a bit of water if necessary to cover the bottom of the pan. Many people learn to use no fat at all, and just simmer their onions, etc., in water until translucent.

For stuffings, sauces, and gravies, use water, dry wine, or vegetable or meat bouillon in place of butter and cream. For example, many rich stuffings for fish and fowl call for as much as a quarter of a cup of butter and a quarter of a cup of heavy cream, which contain a total of 600 calories. These recipes will taste just as good with a tablespoon of butter for flavor, and a fifty–fifty mixture of water and white wine, or bouillon and white wine, and the calorie total will be 100 to 150. Low-fat milk can be substituted for cream in many recipes (12 vs. 100 calories per ounce).

When making meat sauces for pasta and casseroles, be sure to cook the ground beef so that you can press it and pour off any excess fat before combining it with the other ingredients. In this way you will save between 200 and 400 calories per pound of meat. Of course, you should use extra-lean meat to begin with.

Our own dessert recipes are compromises with this Spartan approach. Ordinarily, for example, a kuchen might call for a cup of heavy cream and a cup of sugar (1200 calories, total) mixed with the layer of fruit. We will make this with sour cream or half and half (60 and 40 calories to the ounce, respectively, in comparison with that 100 for heavy cream). Sugar is reduced by 25 percent. This saves either 320 or 480 calories in fat and another 200 in sugar. Then, instead of using half a cup of butter and two cups of flour for the crust (about 1600 calories) we use zwieback and save over 1100 calories in that part of the recipe alone. In the end, one piece contains about 125 calories instead of the 250 in the original recipe.

We have prepared this recipe with many different fruits and it is a smash at our best dinner parties. Give it a try and then use the principles in your own desserts. The recipe is on page 199.

Guidelines for Sandwiches

Many people shy away from bread and other "starches" because they have the mistaken idea that they are particularly high in calories and make it harder to lose weight. The truth is that most breads have about 70 calories per slice, so it is quite easy to make a nutritious, low-calorie luncheon sandwich.

As your basic sandwich recipe I suggest you use:

Two slices of bread

Plus two slices of cheese, sliced lean meat, or fowl

or

3 oz. of tuna or salmon

or

Up to 3 oz. of one of my spreads (p. 161)

plus

1 t. of mayonnaise if you like,

and just about all the mustard or

catsup you want

with

Loads of bean sprouts, or lettuce,

and a couple of slices of
tomato on the sandwich itself.

If that isn't quite enough, you can add an assortment of raw vegetables on the side, and it will still be rather hard to eat over 350 calories.

When you make an open-face sandwich (one slice of bread), use about half the spread, tuna, or salmon, and there will be plenty of room for the cup of soup and other luncheon suggestions on my daily menus. You will not end up with over 300 to 350 calories for the total meal.

A Word on Snacks

Use fresh fruits and vegetables (List I, p. 140) for snacks. Substitute these natural foods for the processed variety (chips and candy) or at the times you might have had a diet drink. If you are thirsty, try an apple or an orange followed by a glass of water. Or drink real unsweetened fruit juices. You will be better nourished and less hungry the rest of the day or night.

I almost always have an apple each day, and several other pieces of fruit from the great variety we keep in the house. We are never without oranges and grapefruit of the easy-to-peel-and-section varieties, grapes, bananas, melons, cherries, pineapple, and berries in season. I occasionally splurge on mangoes, papaya, and kiwi fruit when they are not ridiculously priced, as they tend to be in Nashville.

I usually keep on my desk a glass of ice water containing a slice of lemon or lime to sip on.

While I prefer fruits for snacking, I find that tender yellow summer squash, carrot sticks, and celery are also satisfying.

But don't neglect good whole-wheat bread as a snack—it's far better for you than that package of snack crackers or chips that you find in the vending machines. Carry a chunk of whole-wheat bread with you to work, or see my recipes (pp. 202–04), as well as fruit. Good bread needs nothing on it for nibbling.

While it is not high in fiber, a glass of low-fat milk is an excellent snack if, in that way, you assure yourself of an adequate intake of calcium. Why not have it with a bowl of cereal?

If you choose foods wisely, as I suggest, there is never a need to go hungry. In the end, the more often you eat, nibbling and snacking in between meals, the fewer total calories you may ingest, especially when you substitute more natural foods for the DC processed variety.

Salads

Antipasto

1 medium green pepper, sliced	16 fresh mushrooms
1 Bermuda onion, thinly sliced	Several leaves of leaf lettuce or romaine
12 asparagus spears, cooked or canned	1 6½-oz. can water-pack tuna, drained and flaked
1 cup lightly cooked celery sticks	2 hard-boiled eggs, sliced
1 large tomato, sliced	Chopped parsley for garnish
1 medium cucumber, sliced	3 T. Vinaigrette Dressing (p. 160)

Marinate onion and pepper overnight in 1 T. Vinaigrette Dressing. Sprinkle 2 T. dressing on asparagus, celery, tomatoes, cucumber, and mushrooms, and refrigerate at least 2 hours before serving. Place lettuce or romaine on serving dish and arrange other ingredients. Top with tuna and sliced eggs. Garnish with parsley and sprinkle the marinade remaining from the earlier steps over the salad. Variations: substitute sardines, shrimp, crabmeat, or canned salmon for the tuna.
Serves 4.

Creative Chef Salad

Variety in a fresh vegetable salad is limited only by your imagination. Experiment with different dressings as well as vegetables.
Here is a simple one for starters:

Several large leaves of lettuce or romaine	1 egg quartered (optional)
	1 tomato, quartered
¼ head any favorite lettuce, shredded	1 slice of green pepper
	1 radish rosette
¼ cup red cabbage, shredded	1 T. your favorite dressing (p. 158)
¼ cup shaved carrots	
1 oz. Swiss cheese, cut in narrow strips	Herb Salt (p. 206) to taste
	Freshly ground black pepper to taste
1 oz. white meat of chicken or turkey, in strips	

Arrange green leaves on large serving dish or bottom of a serving bowl. Cover with shredded lettuce, followed by cabbage and carrots. Arrange cheese and chicken in an attractive pattern, with tomato wedges and egg around the sides. Place the slice of green pepper and the radish smack in the middle and sprinkle with dressing.

This is a pretty hefty salad for one person, but I get carried away when I put one of these together. Even at that, it only adds up to about 400 calories, including the egg.

Take a look at Vegetable List I (p. 140) for vegetable ideas, and, for variety, substitute shellfish, tuna, sardines, or other cheeses for the Swiss cheese and chicken.

Creative Fruit Salad

Use any combination of fruits you have on hand, cut up into chunks. For an extra touch, add a tablespoon or so of one or more of the following:

Grated coconut	Lemon juice (this also keeps
Chopped nuts, any variety	the fruit looking fresh)
Raisins	

Try adding a sprinkling of one or more of the following spices:

Cinnamon	Ginger
Nutmeg	Anise
Allspice	Cardamom

Egg Salad

2 hard-boiled eggs
1 stalk celery, sliced
2 t. Dijon mustard

Salt and pepper to taste
Mayonnaise

Mash eggs with a fork, add remaining ingredients with just enough mayonnaise to moisten.
Serves 2.

Macaroni Salad

2 cups cooked elbow macaroni
1 (17-oz.) can small peas
2 hard-boiled eggs, chopped

2 stalks celery, chopped
½ green pepper

Dressing:

1 T. olive oil
2 T. lemon juice
3 T. mayonnaise
1 t. Dijon mustard

1 clove garlic
1 medium onion
Salt and pepper to taste

Puree dressing ingredients and combine with remaining items. Chill.
Serves 8–10.

Marinated Mushrooms

1 lb. fresh mushrooms   ¼–⅓ cup Italian dressing

Wash mushrooms and trim stems. Toss with dressing, and let marinate for at least an hour before serving.
Serves 4.

Pepper and Tomato Salad

3 green peppers thinly sliced
3 tomatoes thinly sliced
  Romaine lettuce
2 T. chopped chives
2 T. chopped parsley

Herb Salt (p. 206) to taste
Freshly ground black pepper
  to taste
2 T. Tarragon Vinegar
  Dressing (p. 160)

Alternate slices of pepper and tomato on leaves of romaine. Top with chives and parsley. Sprinkle with dressing and add herb salt and pepper to taste.
    Serves 6.

Piquant Salad

  2 cups romaine, chopped
16 large pitted ripe olives,
    halved
  2 hard-boiled eggs, sliced
  2 tomatoes, sliced
  ½ avocado
  4 pimientos

2 oz. bleu cheese, crumbled
¼ cup chopped parsley
2 T. White Wine Vinegar
  Dressing (p. 160)
or
Vinaigrette Dressing
(p. 160)

Spread romaine on the bottom of a salad bowl and arrange other ingredients on top in an attractive pattern. Chill. Sprinkle dressing just before serving.
    Serves 4.

Sliced Tomatoes and Cucumbers

2 medium tomatoes, sliced
1 medium cucumber, sliced
1 T. Tarragon Vinegar
  Dressing (p. 160)

Herb Salt (p. 206) to taste
Freshly ground black pepper
  to taste

Mix vegetables with seasonings and allow to marinate in the refrigerator for at least an hour before using.
    This snappy salad goes well with almost any main course, and you can use it for lunch, served on leaves of lettuce or romaine, with a slice of bread and cheese.
    Serves 4.

Stuffed Zucchini Salad

6 medium zucchini squash	Herb Salt (p. 206) to taste
1 can sardines	Freshly ground black pepper
1 t. lemon juice	to taste
3 hard-boiled eggs, diced	¼ cup Parmesan cheese
2 tomatoes, chopped	2 T. chopped parsley for
1 T. parsley	garnish

Boil whole zucchini in small amount of water until just tender. Cut in half lengthwise, scoop out insides, and chop and mash. Drain and mash sardines. Mix with mashed squash and add lemon juice. Season with herb salt and pepper. Stuff shells and cover with diced hard-boiled eggs and tomatoes.

Refrigerate at least 2 hours before serving. Pour about 1 T. Tarragon Vinegar Dressing (p. 160) over each, or use your own favorite dressing. Excellent luncheon dish served on greens, or use as a side dish for dinner.

Serves 3 for lunch, or makes 6 small salads for dinner.

Tossed Salad

About ½ head of your favorite greens added to a small portion of other thinly sliced or diced vegetables makes your basic tossed dinner salad for four.

For each person, add:

½ carrot, thinly sliced	¼ cup shredded red cabbage
1 stalk celery, thinly sliced	or
or	4 sliced mushrooms
¼ green pepper, diced	2 thin slices sweet red onion

Figure about ½ T. of your favorite dressing (p. 158) per person, and add Herb Salt (p. 206) and freshly ground black pepper to taste.

Tuna (or Salmon) Salad

1 6½-oz. can water-pack tuna	2 stalks celery, sliced
(or salmon)	10 pimiento stuffed olives
1 large carrot, sliced	

Blend in food processor or blender, adding enough salad dressing or mayonnaise for desired consistency. Serve with lettuce and tomato for salad, or as a sandwich with sprouts.

Makes two salad portions, or four sandwiches.

Salad Dressings

These recipes for salad dressings vary from no calories (No-Cal Vinegar Dressing) to approximately 65 calories (Red Wine Vinegar) per tablespoon. When using an oil and vinegar formula, figure a half to one tablespoon for an average dinner-salad-size serving. Do the same with commercial dressings. When eating out, order dressing on the side, since many restaurants think nothing of dumping a quarter cup or more of dressing on a chef's salad.

Red Wine Vinegar

4 oz. fine olive oil
2 oz. red wine vinegar
1 t. Dijon mustard
Fresh or dried salad herbs, to
  taste (e.g., ¼ t. each of
  dried basil, thyme,
marjoram, and oregano,
plus a few sprigs of
rosemary, and 1 T. fresh
chopped parsley)
Salt and freshly ground black
  pepper to taste

Place oil in vinegar in jar, add mustard, and mix. Add herbs and seasonings, cover jar, and shake well to blend. Refrigerate. It will last at least 2 weeks. If oil separates when chilled, allow to warm for a few minutes before use and shake well.

Variations: a clove of crushed garlic, 1 T. minced onion, or a pinch of cayenne pepper.

For a thinner dressing, add 4 oz. water (equal amounts water and oil if you change quantity).

Mustard and Mayonnaise

Blend 1 part Dijon mustard to 3 parts mayonnaise. For variety, add a pinch of tarragon to each tablespoon of the mixture.

This simple dressing is excellent with cold fish and all greens. It make a good seasoning for sandwiches, spread thinly.

Tangy Yogurt Mustard Dressing

2 oz. Dijon mustard
1 oz. white vinegar
2 oz. yogurt
¼ cup chopped dill or parsley

Herb Salt (p. 206) to taste
Freshly ground black pepper
to taste

Blend well. Will keep 2 weeks in refrigerator. Use with seafood and vegetables.

Buttermilk Dressing

4 oz. buttermilk
4 oz. cottage cheese
1 t. minced onion

1 clove garlic, crushed
1 t. lemon juice
Herb Salt (p. 206) to taste

Mix in blender. Refrigerate. Will store for a week.

Green Herb Dressing

¼ cup fresh parsley
¼ cup fresh watercress
4 scallions
1 t. dry mustard
2 oz. water
2 oz. salad oil

2 oz. white wine vinegar
½ t. dried tarragon
½ t. choice of mixed salad
herbs
½ t. prepared horseradish

Mix in blender. Very good with greens and seafood.

No-Cal Vinegar Dressing

4 oz. wine vinegar
½ t. Herb Salt (p. 206)
1 T. fresh chopped parsley

1 clove garlic, crushed, or ¼
t. garlic powder

Mix well. Use other herbs to taste for variety.

Vinaigrette Dressing

4 oz. salad oil
1 oz. vinegar
1 oz. lemon juice
1 t. dry mustard

4 oz. water
Herb Salt (p. 206) to taste
Freshly ground black pepper
   to taste

Blend mustard with small amount of vinegar and then place all ingredients in a jar and shake well. For variety, add other herbs, garlic, or minced onions.

Tarragon Vinegar Dressing

4 oz. fine olive oil
2 oz. wine vinegar
1 clove garlic, crushed

½ t. salt
1 t. dried tarragon

Blend by shaking well in a jar, and let stand for several hours before using.

Use with cold Stuffed Zucchini Salad (p. 157) and other green salads. Use it for marinating onions and green peppers. Try it if you have been avoiding these vegetables in your salads because they give you indigestion.

White Wine Vinegar Dressing

4 oz. salad oil
2 oz. white wine vinegar
1 t. lemon juice
1 clove garlic, crushed

Herb Salt (p. 206) to taste
Freshly ground black pepper
   to taste

Shake in jar to blend. Special with Piquant Salad (p. 156).

Cottage Cheese Dressing

½ cup cottage cheese
½ cup yogurt
½ green pepper, chopped
4 radishes, sliced

2 T. chives
1 T. poppy seeds
Herb Salt (p. 206) to taste

Mix in blender or food processor.

Cottage cheese and yogurt can be a base for a variety of dressings: try adding ¼ cup cider vinegar, or a small onion or a few scallions, or 2 hard-boiled eggs, or ½ cup bleu cheese.

Excellent with salads and baked potatoes.

See also Cottage Cheese Spread (p. 163).

Spreads

You can create your own tasty spreads for sandwiches, canapés, and salads with a blender or food processor. Variety is limited only by your imagination. Leftovers—meats, beans, vegetables—all can form the base of a spread or salad mixture. To obtain desirable consistency, add small amounts of salad dressing, yogurt, catsup, or mustard, depending upon what seems appealing.

Spreads go well with bread and soup. Use as open-face sandwiches, with one slice of bread. Try the Bean Spread on whole-wheat bread, broiled in the oven with a slice of cheddar cheese and/or a slice of tomato on top, sprinkled with a few herbs.

Here are a few favorites.

Meat Spread

½ lb. cooked meat or fowl
1 small onion, diced
¼ cup wheat germ (or cooked red beans)

2 T. soy flour
Herb Salt (p. 206) to taste
Freshly ground black pepper to taste

Blend all ingredients in food processor. Moisten as needed with salad dressing or catsup. About 1¼ cups.

Clam Spread

1 6½-oz. can minced clams,
    drained
1 cup cottage cheese

3 T. yogurt
¼ t. Herb Salt (p. 206)
1 small onion, diced

Blend all ingredients.
Makes about 2 cups.

Crab Meat Spread

1 cup crab meat
1 stalk celery (with leaves),
    chopped
1 small onion, diced

½ green pepper, diced
1 cup sprouts
1 cup cottage cheese
  Herb Salt (p. 206) to taste

Blend with enough salad dressing to moisten.
Makes about 3 cups.

Vegetable Spread

1 head lettuce, cut up
1 small onion, diced
3 stalks celery, sliced
1 cucumber, cut up

1 green pepper, cut up
2 hard-boiled eggs
  Herb Salt (p. 206) to taste

Moisten with enough salad dressing to blend in food processor.
Makes 3 cups.

This spread can be served as a salad on greens, will go with tuna, salmon, or cottage cheese in a more elaborate salad, and can stuff tomatoes.

Vegetable spreads can be made with just about any combination of vegetables that appeal to your taste. Use salad dressing to moisten, add a bit of soy flour if you like the consistency it will give, and use Herb Salt for flavoring.

Cottage Cheese Spread

½ lb. cottage cheese
¼ t. celery seed
¼ t. dill seed
¼ t. caraway seed
¼ t. Herb Salt (p. 206)

1 T. fresh parsley, chopped
1 small onion, diced
2 T. soy flour (optional)
3 T. wheat germ (optional)

Blend, adding seasoning to taste. Use also as a salad on greens, with your favorite dressing (p. 158) or a dab of yogurt or sour cream. See also Cottage Cheese Dressing (p. 161).

Bean Spread

1 can dark-red kidney beans, drained
1 small onion, sliced
3 T. catsup

⅛ t. cayenne pepper
Herb Salt (p. 206) to taste
Freshly ground black pepper to taste

Blend in food processor, adding catsup if needed. For a tasty open-face sandwich, broil with cheese and sliced tomato, sprinkled with oregano.

Other legumes give different flavors and consistencies. Try light-red beans and chickpeas for variety.

Soups

Don't neglect soup in your Nutrition Plan. People who have soup for lunch tend to weigh less than people who don't! You can substitute soup, an open-face sandwich, and assorted raw vegetables for any lunch.

Here are some of my favorite hot and cold soups.

Bean Soup

1 cup dried beans (kidney, red, lima, pinto) or lentils	1 15-oz. can stewed tomatoes (2 cups fresh, chopped)
4 cups bouillon	¼ cup brown rice or millet
1 large onion with 3 cloves embedded	½ t. ground sage
	1 t. caraway seeds
2 T. butter or salad oil	3 T. fresh chopped parsley
1 onion, sliced	Herb Salt (p. 206) to taste
1 large carrot, thinly sliced	Freshly ground pepper to taste
2 stalks celery, sliced	

Wash beans and soak overnight with onion stuck with cloves in bouillon.

In large pot, sauté sliced onion, celery, and carrots in butter until onion is translucent.

Add broth, beans, and whole onion (remove cloves) to pot. Add remaining ingredients. Cover and simmer gently until done. Beans vary in the amount of cooking they require, so this can take from 1 to several hours. But don't be concerned—the longer you cook soups of this kind, the better. Just simmer on the lowest heat possible. The soup will also improve for days in the refrigerator. We freeze half of our recipes for seconds weeks later.

Serve with grated cheese. Serves 8.

Cold Broccoli Soup

1 head broccoli, leaves and all, cut into small pieces	8 oz. mushrooms, cut into chunks
4 cups bouillon	1 cup of low-fat milk
1 onion, chopped	3 T. sour cream
1 T. butter	Salt and pepper to taste
1 clove garlic, chopped	

Cook broccoli in bouillon until just tender. Cook onion in butter until translucent. Add garlic and stir for about 1 minute. Add mushrooms and cover pan. Cook until mushrooms are barely done, stirring occasionally. Puree all in food processor. Add milk, sour cream, and salt and pepper. Stir until well combined. Chill. Stir before serving. Serves 8–10.

Cold Cauliflower Soup

1 head cauliflower, cubed	3 T. plain yogurt
1 medium onion, cubed	1 cup whole milk
1 large clove garlic, cubed	1 T. chopped chives
4 cups bouillon	Salt and pepper to taste
4 T. sour cream	

Bring bouillon to a boil. Add cauliflower, onion, and garlic and cook until tender. Puree with sour cream and yogurt in blender. Add milk, chives, salt, and pepper. Chill and serve in mugs.

Serves 10.

Cucumber Yogurt Soup

2 cups yogurt	(2 t. dried leaves)
1 cucumber, sliced	Herb Salt (p. 206) to taste
2 t. lemon juice	Freshly ground black pepper
2 cups cold water	to taste
¼ cup fresh mint	

Mix yogurt, cucumber, lemon juice, and dried mint in food processor until smooth. (Blend fresh mint by hand.) Season and chill. Serve cold with a few slices cucumber on top, or another dab of yogurt or sour cream.

Makes four 1-cup servings.

Curried Yogurt Soup

1 cup beef bouillon	½ to 1 t. curry powder
1 cup yogurt	Chopped cucumber, celery,
½ clove garlic, crushed (or	or chives for garnish
garlic powder to taste)	

Blend ingredients except for garnish in food processor and chill. Will keep for a week in the refrigerator.

Add garnish when serving.

Makes four ½-cup servings.

Variations: replace curry with 1 cup greens, 1 tomato, or 1 to 2 T. minced onion.

Egg Flower Soup

4 cups chicken stock
1 T. beef or chicken bouillon
   granules
1 T. ground sesame seeds

1 T. chopped chives
3 eggs, lightly beaten
Dash ginger
Salt and pepper to taste

Place stock in kettle on high heat. Add bouillon, sesame seeds, and chives. Bring to a boil. Remove from heat and slowly pour eggs in, stirring slightly. Add seasonings and serve.
Serves 8.

Gazpacho

4 cups bouillon
2 cups tomato juice
2 T. lemon juice
1 T. oil (optional)
2 cloves garlic
1 green pepper, sliced
1 medium onion, sliced

1 t. each of your favorite herbs
   (e.g., chives, parsley, basil,
   thyme, tarragon, chervil,
   etc.—use about 1 T. fresh)
1 tomato, chopped
1 cucumber, diced
Salt and pepper to taste

Blend garlic, green pepper, onion, and herbs with 1 cup bouillon in food processor until smooth. Mix together thoroughly with remaining ingredients and chill. Serve very cold.
Serves 8.

Greens Soup

¼ cup chopped raw greens
2 T. chopped watercress
1 T. chives
2 T. chopped parsley
4 chopped scallions

2 cups chicken broth
Herb Salt (p. 206) to taste
Freshly ground black pepper
   to taste

Mix ¼ cup broth with greens, watercress, chives, parsley, and scallions in blender or food processor. Add to rest of broth in medium saucepan. Cover and simmer for about 5 minutes.
Makes four ½-cup servings.

Lentil Soup

6 cups bouillon
1½ cups lentils
2 T. butter or salad oil
2 stalks celery, chopped
1 medium onion, sliced
1 T. celery seed
2 medium carrots, sliced thin
1 15-oz. can stewed

tomatoes, or 2 cups
fresh
1 T. lemon juice
½ t. tarragon
Herb Salt (p. 206) to taste
Freshly ground black
pepper to taste

Wash lentils and soak overnight just covered with broth.

In large saucepan, sauté onions and celery in butter until onions are translucent. Add lentils with all of the bouillon, cover, and simmer until tender (about 45 minutes).

For a thick soup, remove lentils at this point, and puree with a small amount of liquid in food processor.

Add remaining ingredients and cook until carrots are tender (15 to 20 minutes).

Serve with strips of sharp cheese in the bottom of each bowl.
Serves 8.

Quick Borscht

1 cup beef bouillon
1 15-oz. can beets and juice
1 medium onion, sliced

1 T. lemon juice
Freshly ground black pepper
to taste

Combine everything in food processor and serve cold with a few slices of cucumber, boiled potato, or a dab of yogurt or sour cream.
Serves 2.

Seafood Gumbo

1 T. butter
1 medium onion, sliced
1 green pepper, sliced
1 cup celery, sliced
1 15½-oz. can stewed tomatoes
3 cups chicken bouillon
1 6½-oz. can tiny shrimp

1 6½-oz. can crabmeat
2 cups okra, fresh or frozen
Herb Salt (p. 206) to taste
Freshly ground black pepper
  to taste
Chopped parsley for garnish

Saute onion, pepper, and celery in butter until onion is translucent. Add broth, tomatoes, crabmeat, shrimp, and okra, and cook for 5 minutes.

Serve sprinkled with parsley. Goes well over brown rice for a complete meal.

Serves 8.

Seafood Soup Creole

1 can (28 oz.) tomatoes
1½ cups tomato puree or
  sauce
1½ cups water
1 cup brown rice, uncooked
1½ t. salt
2 t. thyme
1 t. garlic powder
½ t. crushed red pepper

1 bay leaf
1 large onion, chopped
½ cup green pepper,
  chopped
1 10-oz. package frozen peas
1 15-oz. can garbanzo beans,
  with juice
3 lbs. fish fillets, cut into
  1-inch chunks

In a large kettle, bring to a boil the tomatoes, tomato puree, water, rice, and seasonings. Add the vegetables and let simmer for about 45 minutes, or until the vegetables get tender. Add the fish and let simmer for an additional 10 to 15 minutes, or until fish is cooked.

Serves 12.

Split Pea Soup

2 cups dried peas	Cheesecloth bag containing
8 cups bouillon	30 black peppercorns and
Old bones from chicken (1	20 whole cloves
carcass) or other meat	1 large onion stuck with 3
1 t. salt	cloves
½ t. turmeric	

Wash and soak peas in bouillon overnight, together with the onion stuck with cloves.

If you are in a hurry and do not have time to soak, bring to a boil for 1 minute and let stand for 1 hour.

Remove whole cloves and combine peas and onion with rest of ingredients. Cover and cook slowly until tender (about 1½ hours).

Remove cheesecloth and squeeze contents into soup. Remove bones and, for a thick soup, blend contents in a food processor. If soup is too thick, add more water.

Serve with cheese, lemon wedges, or croutons.

Serves 8.

Vegetable Chowder

Add ½ cup of your favorite vegetables, sliced or diced, to 2 cups of low-fat milk or 2 cups of bouillon plus 1 T. butter. Season with Herb Salt (p. 206) and freshly ground black pepper.

Vegetable suggestions: celery, carrots, onions, summer squash, mushrooms, green beans, green pepper, cooked potatoes (quartered or sliced)

Sauté onions and peppers first, until onions are translucent. Add remaining ingredients, cover, and simmer 5 to 10 minutes.

Makes four ½-cup servings.

Vichyssoise

This all-time favorite cold soup has one-quarter the calories of the original recipe, which called for 8 T. of butter and 2 cups of heavy cream.

I think you will find this just as tasty as the high-fat recipe.

2 T. butter or salad oil	½ cup powdered low-fat milk
3 leeks, chopped (white parts only)	1 T. soy flour (optional)
1 medium onion, chopped	1 cup yogurt
3 medium potatoes, sliced	1 t. salt (or more to taste at table)
4 cups chicken broth	Chopped chives or scallions
2 cups low-fat milk	for garnish

In large pot, lightly sauté leeks and onions until onions are translucent (add a bit of water if necessary to cover bottom of pot). Do not brown. Add potatoes, broth, and salt. Cover and simmer for 30 minutes.

Remove solids, and with ¼ cup of the liquid, puree in food processor. Return to pot.

Mix soy flour, powdered milk, and milk, and add to pot.

Cover and bring to the edge of a boil. Stop cooking at this point and refrigerate. At time of serving, blend in the yogurt, and serve very cold with chives or scallions.

Serves 8.

Watercress Soup

1 cup watercress	2 scallions, chopped
2 cups chicken broth	Herb Salt (p. 206) to taste

Blend ¼ cup broth with watercress and scallions in food processor. Combine with rest of broth in medium saucepan and bring to near boil. Simmer for 1 minute. Serve hot or cold with slice of lemon.

Makes four ½-cup servings.

Main Courses

Almond Chicken

3 lbs. chicken breasts, skinned and deboned	½ cup whole-wheat flour
⅓ cup soy sauce	½ cup finely ground almonds
1 t. ground ginger	½ t. salt
1 t. garlic powder	½ t. pepper
	2 T. peanut or corn oil

In a large bowl combine the soy sauce, ginger, and garlic powder. Cut the chicken into bite-size chunks and marinate it in the soy sauce mixture while you prepare the other ingredients.

In another bowl, combine flour, almonds, and the rest of the seasonings. Add this to chicken and toss gently until the chicken is coated with the flour mixture.

Heat the oil in a wok or large saucepan on high heat. When the oil is hot, add the chicken, and turn the heat down to medium. Cook covered, stirring often, until the chicken is cooked (about 20 minutes). This is good served with rice and a green vegetable.

Serves 8.

Artichoke Casserole

2 T. butter	2 well-beaten eggs
2 T. whole-wheat flour	2 cans (14 oz. each) artichoke hearts
1 cup skim milk	
1 finely chopped onion	¼ t. paprika
1 cup cheddar cheese, grated	Salt and pepper to taste

Melt butter. Stir in flour and brown gently for a couple of minutes. Add milk, onion, cheese, and seasonings. Pour one can of artichokes and liquid into blender, and puree. Add to saucepan. Drain the other can of artichokes, and add them to the saucepan.

Cook on low about 30 minutes until hot. Do not boil.

Remove from heat and add eggs. Pour into casserole dish, sprinkle with paprika, and bake, covered, for 40 minutes at 350 degrees. Remove cover and bake 5 more minutes.

This can also be served by simply eliminating baking it in the oven. Just spoon it from the saucepan over cooked grain.

Serves 6.

Baked Pork Chops with Caraway Seeds

6 one-inch-thick chops (or 3
   lbs. pork tenderloin, cut
   into 6 pieces)
2 cloves garlic, chopped (or
   garlic powder to taste)

1 t. caraway seeds
2 t. paprika
1 cup dry white wine
   Salt and pepper to taste

Mix together the dry ingredients, as well as the garlic, and rub into chops or tenderloin. Place in large casserole and add wine. Marinate for at least 2 hours in the refrigerator.

Preheat oven to 300 degrees. Bake, uncovered in marinade, for 75 to 90 minutes, or until tender, adding more wine if necessary. This dish goes well with a baked potato, noodles, or rice. Serve with the sauce from the pan.

Serves 6.

Baked Salmon in Foil

This dish deserves special treatment and usually gets it in every cookbook.

The present highly satisfactory version was born out of necessity —I had 10 minutes to prepare it before I had to leave the house for an appointment.

1 3½- to 4-pound fresh salmon
½ t. each: celery seed, tarragon, marjoram, basil, thyme leaves, and a few sprigs of rosemary

Salt, freshly ground pepper, garlic, and onion powder to taste
1 oz. lemon juice
¾ cup water

Wash fish and place it in heavy-duty foil in large baking dish.

Sprinkle salt, pepper, garlic, and onion powder on both sides of fish.

Sprinkle herbs on both sides of fish.

Cover with lemon juice and water.

Fold over ends of foil to cover fish completely and squeeze together well so that liquid will not boil away.

Cook at 375 degrees about 15 minutes per pound. Test fish with tines of a fork; it will flake nicely when done.

To serve, dip out fish bouillon from the foil and heat in another pan. Correct seasonings with water if necessary. Place bouillon in heated serving bowl, and let each person use as desired.

A tangy rémoulade can be made with 1 cup mayonnaise, 2 t. Dijon mustard, 1 t. lemon juice, and 1 t. tarragon leaves. Mix well and let it stand in the refrigerator at least 1 hour before serving. Use sparingly, and save the remainder for sandwiches and salads. It will also go well with cold fish the next day.

Serves 6–8.

Baked Trout (or Fish Fillets)

4 small trout (rainbow, about ¾ lb. each) or 1 lb. fish fillets
1 T. oil

Herb Salt (p. 206) to taste
Freshly ground black pepper to taste

Preheat oven to 500 degrees. Pour oil onto aluminum-lined baking pan, swish fish around well, season, and bake for about 12 minutes, or until fish flakes easily with a fork.

You may broil the fish if you prefer.

Serves 4.

Cabbage Rolls

1 cup brown rice
2 cups beef broth
1 onion, sliced
1 lb. ground veal
1 large head of cabbage
¼–½ t. sage
¼ t. marjoram
Salt and pepper to taste

1 (28 oz.) can tomato puree
1 bay leaf
1 t. basil
½ t. marjoram
1 (28 oz.) can whole tomatoes

Cook rice in broth with onion. Brown veal, and drain fat. Mix rice with veal, sage, marjoram, salt, and pepper.

Parboil cabbage in water to cover until just barely tender.

Peel cabbage leaves off and place a couple teaspoons of veal mixture on the edge of each leaf. Fold leaf over once, then fold in edges to seal the ends, and roll up the rest of the leaf. Fasten with toothpicks.

Place the cabbage rolls in a large kettle in which you have put the tomato puree and remaining seasonings. Top with the whole tomatoes.

Bring to a boil, then let simmer for 1½ to 2 hours, until cabbage is cooked well.

Serves 8.

Cauliflower Italian Style

20 oz. frozen cauliflower	1 cup grated cheddar cheese
½ cup water	1 t. basil
1 clove garlic, chopped fine	½ t. onion powder
1 (28 oz.) can tomato puree	Salt and pepper to taste

Cook cauliflower in water until just tender. Add remaining ingredients and simmer until hot, and cauliflower is cooked through.

Serve over rice.

4 servings.

Cheddar Chili Pie

1 lb. lean ground beef, or veal	2 T. chili powder
1 large onion (or four green onions), chopped	1 t. cumin
2 cloves garlic, chopped fine	¼ t. cayenne
1 can (28 oz.) tomatoes	½ t. crushed red pepper
1 can (15 oz.) kidney beans, with juice	½ t. black pepper
1¼ cups cornmeal	Dash Tabasco sauce
1 cup grated cheddar cheese	1¼ cups skim milk
	2 eggs, lightly beaten
	Salt and pepper to taste

Sauté beef, onion, and garlic until brown. Drain off fat. Add tomatoes, beans, ¾ cup cornmeal, ½ cup cheese, and the seasonings. Cook over low heat, stirring occasionally, for about 15 minutes. Pour into casserole dish.

In the same pan, combine the milk, the rest of the cornmeal, and the salt and pepper to taste. Stir over low heat until it thickens a little. Then add the remaining cheese and the eggs, stirring until smooth. Pour this over the ground-beef mixture. Bake uncovered at 375 degrees for 30 minutes or until crust is lightly browned.

Serves 6.

Chicken with Broccoli

1 T. oil
1 large clove garlic, minced
3 lbs. chicken breasts, skinned
    and deboned
⅓ cup dry sherry
¼ to ½ cup soy sauce

2 T. cornstarch
¼ cup cold water
½ t. ground ginger
1 bunch fresh broccoli, cut
    into slender pieces

Cut chicken into chunks. Heat oil in wok or large saucepan on medium heat. Add garlic and stir-fry 1 minute. Add chicken; stir-fry until browned.

Add remaining ingredients. Cook covered, stirring occasionally for 40 minutes or until broccoli is tender.

Serve over rice or another grain.

Serves 6–8.

Crab Quiche with Crumb Topping
(Makes 2)

2 packages frozen crabmeat
2 cups skim milk
2 cups grated cheddar cheese
6 eggs
2 t. dried parsley
½ t. salt
¼ t. pepper

¼ t. marjoram
¼ t. garlic powder
¼ t. nutmeg
2 cups Pepperidge Farm
    seasoned bread crumbs
½ T. butter

Layer the crab in the bottoms of two empty pie pans.

Combine all other ingredients except bread crumbs and butter, and pour half of mixture into each pie pan.

Bake at 350 degrees for 30 minutes. Then top each quiche with 1 cup of bread crumbs and dot with ¼ T. butter. Bake 15 minutes more.

Cut into slices and serve.

8 servings.

Crab with Vermicelli

2 six-oz. packages frozen crabmeat, thawed, with liquid
1 T. butter
2 cloves garlic, chopped fine
½ t. marjoram
½ cup chopped green onion
½ cup white wine
2 t. parsley flakes
Sprinkling of rosemary leaves
Salt and pepper to taste

Melt butter in frying pan over medium heat. Add spices and green onion and sauté until transparent. Stir in remaining ingredients. Simmer gently until crab is heated. Serve over vermicelli (or rice if you prefer).

Serves 4.

Fillet of Lemon Sole with Almonds

1½ lbs. lemon sole fillets
1 T. oil
1 T. lemon juice
1 T. chopped almonds
A few pinches of dried
parsley
1 half of a lemon
Salt
Pepper

In the bottom of a shallow baking pan, spread the oil, lemon juice, and salt and pepper to taste. Swish the fish around in the pan, coating both sides with the oil mixture. Then sprinkle on top the almonds and the parsley. Squeeze the juice of the half lemon over the top.

Broil 3½ minutes on each side under high heat, about 1½ inches from the heat, or until the edges are browned.

Serves 4.

Fillet of Sole Florentine

2 cups chicken broth
4 T. whole-wheat flour
2 cloves garlic, chopped fine
2 packages frozen spinach,
    thawed and drained

Thyme
2 lbs. sole fillets
2 ounces grated Parmesan
    cheese
Paprika

In frying pan on low heat, combine chicken broth, flour, and garlic. Stir occasionally until thickened. Spoon a thin layer into each of two 9 × 11 inch shallow baking dishes. Spread a layer of spinach on top of the broth mixture. Sprinkle with thyme. Arrange a layer of fish over the spinach. Pour the rest of the broth over this. Sprinkle with cheese and paprika.

Bake uncovered at 400 degrees for about 30 minutes, or until fish is flaky.

Serves 8.

Fish Roll-ups

2 lbs. fish fillets
2 T. tomato paste
2 T. Dijon mustard
6 T. yogurt
1 onion

1 large clove garlic
1 green pepper, julienned
Pepper
Chives

Sprinkle each fillet with chives and pepper. Put about 1 T. of green pepper on each. Then roll up and skewer each one. Place them in a baking dish.

Puree remaining ingredients in food processor and pour over fish. Bake in preheated 350-degree oven for 45 minutes or until fish flakes easily with a fork, basting occasionally.

Serves 8.

Lemon-Baked Chicken

About 7 lbs. chicken pieces, skinned	½ t. thyme
½ cup lemon juice	½ t. marjoram
2 onions, cut into chunks	½ t. pepper
½ t. garlic powder	¼ t. rosemary
	2 t. dried parsley

Combine all ingredients in a large casserole dish and marinate, covered in the refrigerator, for at least an hour, stirring occasionally.

Preheat oven to 350 degrees and bake chicken for about an hour and a half.

Serves 8–10.

Marinated Flank Steak

Here are two interesting and quite different marinades for flank steak and other meats. They can be used for outdoor grilling as well.

1 T. salad oil	⅛ t. thyme leaves
½ cup dry white wine	1 bay leaf
2 large cloves garlic, minced	1 t. chives
1 small onion, minced	2 lbs. lean flank steak

Marinate steak overnight in covered bowl, or double plastic Baggies.

Broil 4 minutes to a side, basting with marinade as you turn. Use all the marinade. Slice thinly on the diagonal to serve, and cover with sauce from the pan. Add salt and freshly ground black pepper at the table if desired.

An oriental marinade:

1 T. salad oil	peeled and grated (or minced). (You can
¼ cup soy sauce	substitute ¼ to ½ t.
¼ cup red wine	powdered ginger, but it is
4 cloves garlic, minced	far from the same flavor
4 scallions, minced	as fresh root.)
4 whole peppercorns	
1-inch cube of ginger,	

Marinate overnight and cook as above.

Serves 8.

Oven-Fried Catfish

1 lb. catfish fillets (or substitute other fish)	¼ t. salt
	¼ t. paprika
2 T. skim milk	¼ t. onion powder
1 egg	½ to 1 t. oil
½ cup yellow cornmeal	1 T. butter

Preheat oven to 500 degrees. Beat milk and egg together in one bowl, and combine in another shallow bowl or plate the cornmeal and seasonings.

Dip each fish fillet into the egg and then into the cornmeal mixture, coating fillets thoroughly.

Coat a shallow baking dish with the oil, and place the fish in a single layer in the baking dish. Dot the fillets with the butter.

Bake for about 12 minutes, or until flaky.

Serves 4.

Poached Eggs Italian Style

1 (28 oz.) can tomato puree	½ cup water
3 rounded T. tomato paste	8 eggs
1 t. basil	Salt and pepper to taste
1 t. oregano	3 T. grated Parmesan cheese
½ t. garlic powder	8 slices whole-wheat toast
½ t. onion powder	

Heat tomato puree, paste, basil, oregano, garlic, onion powder, and water in a large shallow saucepan. When it just comes to a boil, break eggs gently into sauce, season with salt and pepper, and poach for about 5 minutes. Sprinkle with cheese and let simmer until cheese melts.

Serve over toast.

4 servings.

Rice and Beans

Beans:

2 cups dried beans, rinsed and
  drained
4 or 5 cups bouillon or broth
1 onion, peeled

4 whole cloves
2 dried red peppers
  Salt and pepper to taste
1 bay leaf

Rice:

2 cups rice
4 cups bouillon or broth
1 t. chopped chives

1 t. dried bell peppers
  Salt and pepper to taste

Soak beans overnight in broth along with the onion stuck with 4 cloves and the bay leaf. Next day, add red pepper and bring beans to boil, adding more water as necessary; reduce to simmer and cook 4 or 5 hours until very tender. Season to taste.

Cook rice in bouillon along with chives and green peppers. Season with salt and pepper. Heat beans and ladle over rice portions.

Serves 8.

Sesame Almond Chicken

About 7 lbs. chicken pieces,
  skinned
1 cup bread crumbs or
  Pepperidge Farm stuffing
  mix
½ cup slivered almonds
¼ cup ground sesame seeds

1 clove garlic, chopped fine
½ t. each onion powder,
  thyme, marjoram, salt
1 t. parsley
1 t. dry mustard
¼ t. pepper
1 egg, lightly beaten

Combine dry ingredients and seasonings; mix well. Place a layer of chicken pieces in the bottom of a large casserole dish. Brush the chicken with the beaten egg. Sprinkle with some of the sesame-almond mixture. Continue layering chicken, egg, and sesame-almond mixture until all ingredients are used up.

Bake covered at 300 degrees for 1½ to 2 hours.

Serves 8–10.

Spaghetti with Garlic and Clam Sauce

8 oz. thin spaghetti (try spinach spaghetti or substitute "spinach" spaghetti that is made from Jerusalem artichoke flour—it's delicious with this sauce)
1 T. butter or oil
2 cans (6½ oz.) minced clams, drained (reserve liquid)
2 T. butter or oil
4 large cloves of garlic, minced
¼ cup freshly chopped parsley (2 t. dried)
8 T. freshly grated Parmesan or Romano cheese

Cook spaghetti in plenty of boiling water to which 1 T. oil has been added to prevent sticking.

In 4-quart saucepan, melt 2 T. butter or oil and gently cook garlic until it begins to turn color (do not brown). Add clams and heat 3 minutes; add clam juice and parsley and continue to simmer gently until spaghetti is done.

Drain spaghetti in colander, and then empty it into the saucepan with the clams and garlic. Mix well. Serve with 2 T. (1 oz.) grated cheese per person.

The sauce can be made with 4 oz. dry white wine, but allow it to simmer down. You do not need much liquid for this sauce.

Serves 4.

Spicy Chicken with Lemon and Onions

12 pieces of chicken (breasts, thighs, and drumsticks)
3 medium onions
  1-inch cube of fresh ginger, peeled and coarsely chopped
4 large cloves of garlic, chopped
2 T. salad oil
1 T. ground coriander
1 t. ground cumin
½ t. ground turmeric

2 T. plain yogurt
4 T. tomato sauce
½ t. salt
¼ t. ground cinnamon
¼ t. ground cloves
2 whole dried hot red peppers (or ⅛ t. cayenne)
1 whole lemon
⅛ t. freshly ground black pepper
  Water as indicated below

Skin the chicken (you cannot fully appreciate this dish if you leave the skins on—in fact, you may never again want to eat chicken without skinning it once you have experimented with Indian cooking).

Slice one onion into thin rounds.

Chop two onions coarsely.

Place coarsely chopped onions in blender with 6 T. water, ginger, and garlic. Make a paste.

Heat 2 T. oil in large skillet and lightly brown sliced onions. Remove and drain on paper towels.

Pour paste into skillet, averting eyes. Heat on medium until paste begins to brown. Add red peppers, coriander, cumin, and turmeric, stirring and heating for 2 minutes.

Add yogurt, stirring and heating for 2 minutes; add tomato sauce, stirring and heating for 2 minutes.

Add salt, cinnamon, cloves, and 1½ cups of water. Bring to the edge of a boil, cover, reduce heat, and simmer for 5 minutes.

Cut lemon into thin slices. Add lemon slices, along with chicken, fried onions, and ground black pepper to the skillet.

Bring to the edge of a boil once again and turn down heat. Cover and simmer gently for about 30 minutes, or until chicken is tender. Turn chicken occasionally. Add more water if needed, but end with a thick sauce.

Excellent with any rice dish, boiled or baked potatoes, carrots, peas, cauliflower, or broccoli.

Serves 6.

Spicy Oven-Fried Chicken

6 lbs. chicken pieces	1 t. black pepper
1½ cups flour (whole wheat, white, or combination)	¾ t. onion powder
	¾ t. garlic powder
1 T. paprika	¼–½ t. cayenne
1 t. salt	

Combine flour and seasonings, and dredge each piece of chicken in this mixture. Place the chicken with skin side down on baking sheets. Sprinkle ¾ of the remaining flour mixture over the chicken.

Bake for 30 minutes at 350 degrees. Then turn the chicken pieces over, sprinkle them with the rest of the flour and bake 30 minutes more.

Serves 8–10.

Spinach Pesto and Pasta

1½ cups cottage cheese	½ t. basil
1 clove garlic, chopped	½ t. oregano
10 oz. frozen spinach, thawed and drained	2 green onions (optional)
	1 T. plain yogurt
1 T. dried parsley	Salt and pepper to taste
2 T. grated Parmesan cheese	

Blend all ingredients in blender or food processor.

Cook pasta (vermicelli is good), drain, and spoon pesto over each serving.

Serves 6–8.

Tandoori Chicken

When this rather spicy dish is made in India, it is cooked in a clay oven, open at the top, with a live coal or wood fire blazing inside. The chicken is always skinned, and colored a bright reddish-orange with a vegetable food coloring. I skip the coloring.

I make this dish in a large skillet, or barbecue it over medium-hot coals about 20 minutes per side, brushing it with the marinade as needed.

18 pieces of chicken (breasts, legs, and thighs), skinned	1 t. ground cumin
	1 t. ground turmeric
1 large onion, chopped	¼ t. ground cardamom
4 to 6 whole cloves of garlic, chopped	¼ t. ground mace
	¼ t. ground nutmeg
1 piece of fresh ginger, 1 by 2 inches, peeled and chopped	¼ t. ground cloves
	¼ t. ground cinnamon
	½ t. ground black pepper
3 T. lemon juice	1 t. salt
8 oz. plain yogurt	¼ to ½ t. cayenne pepper (go lightly the first time you use this recipe)
1 T. ground coriander	

Make the marinade by putting the onions, garlic, ginger, and lemon juice in a blender and mixing to a smooth paste (some blenders may require a bit of water added to make adequate contact). Place the mixture in a bowl large enough to hold the chicken, and add the yogurt, salt, and all the spices. Mix thoroughly.

Put the skinned pieces of chicken in the marinade and rub them with the mixture. You will get more penetration if you make a few slashes in each piece of chicken with the point of a sharp knife, but I have not always done this and it tastes fine without going to this extra bother. Marinate overnight in the refrigerator. Again, I have sometimes cut this time down to 2 hours when I am going to use the skillet version, and it works out well.

Skillet cooking: You can empty the entire contents into a large skillet, bring the marinade that covers it to the bare edge of a boil over high heat, and then cover the skillet and reduce heat to a simmer for 45 to 60 minutes. Or, if you like your chicken browned, remove it from the marinade, brown in a small amount of vegetable oil or butter, and then add the marinade and simmer for 45 to 60 minutes.

Barbecue version: Place the pieces of chicken on a grill about 4 to 6 inches above the coals. I don't like my chicken burned, so I let the fire reduce itself just beyond its hottest point before starting the chicken. Baste and turn once or twice during roasting. It will take about 20 minutes per side, or longer, depending upon your fire.

Garnish:

I like this dish served with sliced raw onions that have been marinated in either ice water containing the juice of one lemon, or in Tarragon Vinegar Dressing (p. 160). Slice up enough onions to place a couple of rings over each piece.

And give everyone a lemon wedge or two—a couple of extra drops on each piece will please many people.

Tandoori chicken goes well with almost any vegetable dish. I serve it with Rice and Spinach (p. 195) or baked or boiled potatoes—and extra marinated onions.

Serves 6–8.

Veal and Garbanzos

1 lb. ground veal	½ t. turmeric
2 cloves garlic, minced	½ t. cayenne
1 onion, chopped	1 dried red pepper
1 15-oz. can garbanzo beans	¼ t. ground ginger
1 6-oz. can tomato paste	½ t. Szechuan or red
1 cup plain yogurt	pepper
½ cup skim milk	½ t. salt
¼ t. dry mustard or ground	Pepper to taste
mustard seed	

Brown veal with garlic and onion. Drain off fat. Add remaining ingredients, mixing well, and let simmer until hot. Do not boil. Serve over cooked grain.

Serves 6–8.

Veal Loaf

1 lb. ground veal
1 can (15½ oz.) dark kidney
   beans, drained
½ cup dry bread crumbs
1 egg
2 T. soy sauce
⅛ t. cayenne pepper
1 15-oz. can tomato sauce

1 t. oregano, or 2 T. chopped
   parsley
Dash of Worcestershire
   sauce
Freshly ground black pepper
   to taste

Puree beans in food processor. Remove and add to veal. Blend in bread crumbs, egg, soy sauce, Worcestershire sauce, and black and cayenne peppers, with enough tomato sauce to make a rather smooth consistency (about 3 to 4 T.).

Place in deep baking dish and cover with remaining sauce. Sprinkle with parsley or oregano. If you like your loaves hot, sprinkle a little more cayenne on top of the sauce.

Bake 1 hour at 350 degrees.

You can substitute lean ground beef for veal.

This dish provides an economical and tasty way to stretch meat and still obtain high-quality protein.

Serves 8.

Vegetables

Acorn Squash

Cut in half lengthwise, spoon out seeds, and bake face down on aluminum foil at 350 degrees about 45 minutes or until tender.

For a tasty filling, mix together 2 T. chopped walnuts, pecans, almonds, or any mixed unsalted variety, with 1 medium apple, diced. Halfway through baking, turn squash, fill both halves, and sprinkle with ½ t. brown sugar. Salt to taste at the table.

Serves 2.

Carrot Soufflé

¼ cup water
4 cups carrots, sliced
2 T. butter
¼ cup skim milk
6 T. whole-wheat flour

½ t. salt
½ t. onion powder
2 cups skim milk
6 eggs, separated

Cook carrots in water, drain, and mash. Melt butter in saucepan; add ¼ cup skim milk, flour, and seasonings. Then add the rest of the milk, cooking slowly until thickened.

Beat egg yolks until smooth and add to white sauce, then stir in carrots. Beat egg whites until stiff and fold gently into carrot mixture.

Pour into casserole dish, and set the dish in a pan of hot water in the oven at 350 degrees for 45 to 50 minutes.

Serves 8.

Carrots

3 cups carrots, sliced
1 onion, chopped

Salt, pepper, and parsley to taste
¼ cup water

Place ingredients in saucepan, bring to a boil, and then simmer gently until cooked.

6 servings.

Cauliflower Casserole

1 head cauliflower
½ cup water
1 onion, chopped
1 cup skim milk
2 cups grated cheddar cheese

½ cup mushrooms (canned or fresh)
1½ T. ground sesame seeds
Salt and pepper to taste

Cut the cauliflower into chunks and place in saucepan with water and onion. Bring to a boil and cook until tender. Drain water out. Put cauliflower into a casserole dish along with the rest of the ingredients, mixing well.

Bake covered at 350 degrees for 30 minutes.

Serves 6.

Cauliflower with Mushrooms

10 oz. frozen cauliflower
8 large fresh mushrooms,
   sliced thin
¼ cup water

1 t. dried parsley
Salt, pepper, and onion
   powder to taste
Dash of thyme

Cook cauliflower and mushrooms in water. Add seasonings, simmer a minute more, and serve.

4 servings.

Chana Aur Aloo
(Indian Spiced Chickpeas and Potatoes)

This dish is best when you start from scratch with black or yellow chickpeas, soaked overnight in bouillon together with an onion stuck with 3 or 4 whole cloves. But you can also make it with canned chickpeas (garbanzos) as well, and you might give it a try with the canned variety even if the flavor and texture are rather inferior. If you do not ordinarily use dried beans, I suggest you also give them a try, since the texture is more nutlike and the flavor richer.

1 cup chickpeas (or one 15½-oz. can, drained)
1 medium onion, stuck with 3 or 4 whole cloves
1 medium onion, chopped
1 piece of fresh ginger, about 1 inch square, peeled and diced
3 large cloves of garlic, minced
2 T. vegetable oil or butter
¼ t. whole cumin seeds (use more powder, see below in list, if you cannot find seeds)

4 medium potatoes, quartered
1 t. ground coriander
¼ t. ground turmeric
¼ t. ground cardomom
¼ t. ground black pepper
¼ t. ground cinnamon
⅛ t. ground cloves (¼ if using canned chickpeas)
¼ t. ground cumin (½ if you don't have seeds, above)
⅛ to ¼ t. cayenne pepper (¼ is quite hot)
½ t. salt
2 T. lemon juice

Sort chickpeas, discarding discolored ones, and wash under cold water.

Soak for 24 hours in a bowl with the onion stuck with cloves just covered with bouillon. If you don't have homemade bouillon, use 2 cups of water and 1 heaping teaspoon of dissolved bouillon crystals.

Place chopped onions, garlic, and ginger in blender with 3 T. water and make a smooth paste (use more water if necessary).

In 4-quart saucepan, heat oil or butter and add cumin seeds. They will darken in a few seconds, at which time add the paste from the blender (keep face averted in case of splatter).

Remove cloves from whole onion, and pour in chickpeas and onion with all the remaining bouillon. Add the potatoes and all remaining ingredients except for the lemon juice. If you are using canned chickpeas, add 1 cup water or bouillon.

Bring to a boil, cover, reduce heat, and gently simmer for about an hour. If liquid boils out, add more water to keep bottom of pot covered.

Add lemon juice just before serving and mix well. Sauce should be thick. Check for salt, and add as necessary.

Spicy dishes of this sort are excellent accompaniments to plain cooked fowl, meats, and vegetables. You will find that the flavor livens them up, and makes something like oven-broiled chicken taste quite different from usual.

Sliced tomatoes and cucumbers, plain, in lemon juice, or in Tarragon Vinegar Dressing (p. 160), also make a good accompaniment.

Serves 6–8.

Cooked Carrots with Herbs

8 medium carrots, sliced	¼ t. dill seed
¼ cup water	Herb Salt (p. 206) to taste

Bring water to a boil, and add carrots. Let simmer until just tender. Add the Herb Salt and dill seed, stirring well. Let simmer for another minute or two, and serve.

4 servings.

Green Beans Almondine
(or Green Beans with Mushrooms)

1 10-oz. package frozen green beans	Dash salt
	Dash pepper
¼ cup water	2 T. slivered almonds

Cook green beans in water until tender, add remaining ingredients, and simmer 5 minutes more.

Substitute ¼ cup of mushrooms for the almonds, if desired.

4 servings.

Mushrooms and Peppers à la Grecque

Make the marinade first, then add the vegetables.
Marinade:

1 cup chicken bouillon	2 T. fresh chopped parsley
¼ cup dry white wine	2 T. lemon juice
1 large clove garlic, crushed	1 T. salad oil
or minced	6 peppercorns
1 t. Herb Salt (p. 206)	1 bay leaf

Make a little cheesecloth sack for the peppercorns and bay leaf (or you may want to strain the liquid after cooking instead).

Combine with rest of the ingredients and bring to a boil in a medium saucepan. Reduce heat, cover, and simmer gently for 30 minutes. Remove peppercorns and bay leaf.

Vegetables:

1 lb. fresh mushrooms, halved	red and green) sliced
2 medium onions, quartered	Chopped parsley for garnish
2 green peppers (or 1 each,	

Add onions and peppers to marinade and simmer until just tender. Add mushrooms and simmer 5 minutes more.

Refrigerate overnight and serve cold.

Variation: substitute sliced summer squash for the mushrooms, or add them to the mixture.

This makes a nice lunch with a couple of slices of white-meat chicken, or cold fish.

Serves 4.

Oven-Fried Potato Sticks

4 potatoes	⅛ t. onion powder
1 T. oil	1 to 1½ t. paprika
⅛ t. garlic powder	Salt and pepper to taste

Leave skins on potatoes; slice lengthwise into eighths.

Line a shallow baking pan with foil, and put all ingredients into the pan, tossing well to coat the potatoes with the oil and seasonings.

Bake at 325 degrees for 1 hour, or at a higher temperature for less time if you wish. Adjust seasoning if necessary.

4 servings.

Peas and Baby Onions

1 package (10½ oz.) frozen
    peas, or 1½ cups fresh
1 small can baby onions, or 1
    large onion, sliced

1 T. butter
Herb Salt (p. 206) to taste
Freshly ground pepper to
    taste

Fresh onions should be sautéed first in butter until translucent. Add peas and ¼ cup water and cook until tender.

With canned onions, cook peas first until tender; add onions and butter and warm.

Serve with baked or poached fish.

Serves 4.

Pennsylvania Dutch Potato Pudding

This is my version of an old Pennsylvania Dutch recipe that had a few more calories in it and didn't taste one bit better. I can assure you that it tastes much better than it "reads" and has to be tried to be appreciated.

4 potatoes
4 slices whole-grain
    bread
½ cup milk
½ cup bouillon
1 medium onion, sliced

2 stalks celery, with leaves,
    sliced
1 large carrot, sliced
2 T. butter
Salt and freshly ground
    black pepper to taste

Boil the potatoes, with skins, in salted water.

While the potatoes are boiling, slice the onions, celery, and carrot very thinly (or use your food processor for slicing). Sauté the vegetables in the butter until the onions are translucent. Cut the bread into cubes about ½ to 1 inch in size, and add to the skillet, mixing well with the vegetables.

When the potatoes are done, drain and cut into quarters. Place in large mixing bowl with the sautéed vegetables and bread cubes. Add the milk and bouillon gradually as you mash with an old-fashioned potato masher or large fork. The mixture should be blended well, but leave the potatoes in rather large chunks. Do not even approach the consistency of mashed potatoes.

Add salt and pepper to taste.

Pour into a baking dish and bake for 45 minutes at 350 degrees.

Use any time you would ordinarily serve potatoes.

Serves 8.

Ratatouille

1 medium zucchini, sliced	2 cloves garlic, minced
1 small eggplant, sliced	1 t. Herb Salt (p. 206)
1 medium tomato, sliced	Freshly ground black pepper
1 green pepper, sliced	to taste
1 T. butter or salad oil	Chopped parsley for garnish
1 medium onion, sliced	

Heat butter in a medium saucepan. Add green pepper and onion with a bit of water and sauté until onion is translucent. Add remaining ingredients, cover, and bring to the edge of a boil. Simmer for 5 minutes. Uncover and cook until liquid evaporates. Season to taste. Serve hot, sprinkled with parsley, or cold on greens. A bit of Vinaigrette Dressing (p. 160) goes well with the cold version.

Vary the proportions of vegetables in this dish to suit your taste. You can use several tomatoes and serve it with a stewlike consistency. Try any variety of summer squash. Add a dozen sliced pimiento-stuffed green olives 1 minute before the dish has finished cooking. Or sprinkle with Parmesan cheese.

Serves 4.

Rice

Brown and wild rice, together with other less used grains such as millet and barley, can play a large role in a nutritious diet. I tend to alternate grains such as these with potatoes in my evening meal almost every day.

Basic recipe:

2 cups brown or wild rice	Other seasonings to taste,
1 T. butter or salad oil	such as 1 T. chopped
4 cups bouillon (whatever you	chives, scallions, or Herb
have accumulated in the	Salt (p. 206), depending
freezer from meats, fowl,	on bouillon
and vegetables)	

Melt butter in large saucepan, add rice, and stir until all the grains are coated. This prevents rice from sticking together. Add bouillon, cover, and bring to boil. Reduce heat and simmer gently for 45 minutes, or until all liquid has been absorbed.

Try mixing other grains, such as millet or barley, half and half with rice.

Serves 8.

Rice and Spinach

1 package frozen chopped
    spinach (10½ oz.), or 1
    lb. fresh, trimmed and
    chopped
2 medium onions, peeled and
    chopped
1 T. butter

¼ cup water
1 cup brown or wild rice
2 cups bouillon
⅛ t. each: ground cardamom,
    black pepper, cumin,
    coriander, cinnamon,
    cloves

Melt butter in large saucepan and lightly sauté onions with bit of water until translucent. Add ¼ cup water and spinach, cooking until it is broken up (or the fresh is wilted). Add spices and mix well. Add bouillon and rice, mix well, cover, and bring to boil. Reduce heat and simmer for 45 minutes, or until liquid is absorbed and rice is tender.
    Serves 4.

Seasoned Tomatoes

4 fresh tomatoes
1 to 2 cloves garlic, chopped
    fine
¼ t. tarragon

¼ t. basil
⅛ t. black pepper
1 T. grated Parmesan cheese

Cut tomatoes in half. Place in shallow baking pan, flat side up. Combine seasonings and cheese and sprinkle over tomatoes. Bake at 350 degrees for about 30 minutes, or until tender.
    8 servings.

Snow Peas

1 lb. fresh snow peas
1 T. oil
1 clove garlic, minced
Dash soy sauce

Dash ginger
(Optional: about ¼ to ½ cup
    bouillon and 2 t.
    cornstarch)

Wash and trim ends of snow peas. Heat oil in wok or large saucepan, and fry garlic in oil for about a minute. Add the peas and stir-fry for a few minutes, until evenly coated with oil. Add the soy sauce and ginger. Add the bouillon and cornstarch if you want a sauce. Turn heat down to low, and cover. Simmer gently about 5 to 10 minutes, until peas are just tender, stirring occasionally.
    4 servings.

Spinach and Broccoli Casserole

2 (10-oz.) packages frozen spinach
1 (10-oz.) package frozen broccoli
½ cup water
1 can mushroom soup
½ cup skim milk

½ cup grated Parmesan cheese
½ cup grated cheddar cheese
1 t. each garlic and onion powder
Salt and pepper to taste
1 cup Pepperidge Farm bread crumbs

Cook the spinach and broccoli in the water. Stir in the remaining ingredients. Place in a large casserole dish and top with crumbs. Bake at 350 degrees for 35 to 40 minutes.

Serves 8–10.

Spinach and Other Greens

I like spinach, kale, beet greens, and collards cooked in similar ways. And the stir-fry method can be used as well as boiling or steaming for almost any vegetable, from broccoli, carrots, and celery to zucchini.

Plain, boiled with onions or mushrooms:

Add one medium thinly sliced onion or ½ lb. sliced mushrooms to fresh (1 lb.) spinach or a package frozen.

Always cook greens in smallest possible amount of water, and save liquid for bouillon in the freezer.

Season with Herb Salt (p. 206) and freshly ground pepper to taste. Add 1 T. butter to pot for 4 servings.

Stir-fry:

1 lb. fresh spinach (remove large stems)
1 T. butter or oil
1 medium onion, sliced thin

Herb Salt to taste
Freshly ground black pepper to taste

Wash and drain spinach. Melt butter in skillet and sauté onions for 1 minute. Add spinach and stir until leaves are wilted and the vegetable hot—about 1 minute.

Serve immediately with a squeeze of lemon or a sprinkle of grated cheese.

See also Tomatoes Florentine (p. 197).

Serves 4.

Summer Squash and Onions

6 medium-sized summer
    squash, sliced
1 onion, quartered

1 t. basil
¼ cup water

Bring water to a boil. Add remaining ingredients. Cook until tender, about 15 minutes.
    4 servings.

Tomatoes Florentine

4 large tomatoes
1 package frozen spinach (10
    oz.)
1 T. butter or oil
¼ t. nutmeg

8 t. freshly grated Parmesan
    or Romano cheese
Herb Salt (p. 206) to taste
Freshly ground black pepper
    to taste

Cut tomatoes in half and bake 10 minutes at 350 degrees. Cook spinach in ¼ cup water until tender. Drain (and save broth in freezer for bouillon). Blend spinach with butter, nutmeg, and seasonings in food processor until smooth. Pile mixture on tomato halves, sprinkle 1 t. cheese on each, and return to oven for 15 minutes, or until hot.
    8 servings.

Desserts

Apricot Rice Pudding

½ cup dried apricots	3 eggs, lightly beaten
½ cup raisins	2 cups skim milk
1½ cups rice, or rice and millet combination	1 t. vanilla
	1 t. cinnamon
3 cups combination water and juice from dried fruit (see recipe)	½ t. nutmeg
	½ cup brown sugar

Chop apricots and soak with raisins overnight in water to cover. Drain and reserve juice. Add enough water to juice to make 3 cups. Bring the liquid to a boil. Gradually add the rice. (If millet is used, let the rice cook 15 minutes before adding the millet.)

Turn the heat to low and cook until the grain is tender (about 45 minutes), adding more water if necessary.

Add the dried fruit and let cool. Add the remaining ingredients and pour into a very lightly greased casserole dish.

Bake at 325 degrees for 1 hour. Serve warm or cold. (If this pudding is not sweet enough for your taste, try sprinkling lightly with brown sugar, or ½ t. maple syrup at the table.)

12 servings.

Baked Apples

4 apples	4 t. brown sugar
4 T. raisins	Cinnamon

Wash and core apples, leaving skins on. Place in shallow baking dish. Put a tablespoon of raisins inside each apple, and top with a teaspoon of brown sugar on each apple. Sprinkle with cinnamon, and bake at 350 degrees until tender.

Serves 4.

Baked Honey Custard

4 cups low-fat milk	8 eggs
½ cup honey	1¼ t. ground nutmeg

Place milk in kettle and scald on medium-low heat. Remove from heat, add honey, and let cool while you beat the eggs in a large bowl. Pour milk mixture into eggs. Add nutmeg.

Pour into custard cups or two loaf pans and set the containers in pans of hot water. Bake at 300 degrees for 40 to 50 minutes, until knife inserted in center comes out clean. Serve hot or cold.

Serves 10.

Berry Cream Dessert

1 pint each strawberries and blueberries	1 T. fresh lemon juice
2 eggs, separated	1 t. Cherry Heering or Kirsch
4 T. sugar (6 if you like it really sweet)	

Wash and hull berries. In food processor or blender, combine egg yolks, sugar, lemon juice, and liqueur. Chop berries coarsely in blender or food processor. Beat egg whites until stiff. Combine all ingredients, folding in egg whites last.

Freeze 4 to 6 hours, stirring up from bottom occasionally. This freezes very solid, so take out of the freezer about a half hour before serving.

12 servings.

Blueberry Sour Cream Kuchen

16 zwieback	1 t. cinnamon
1½ pints blueberries	2 eggs
¾ cup brown sugar	1 cup sour cream

Crush zwieback. (I put them in a large, tied baggie, and use a rolling pin.) Pour the crumbs in a 9 × 9-inch square baking pan. Sprinkle half the cinnamon on top, then pour the blueberries on. Top with brown sugar, and place in 400-degree oven for 10 minutes. Meanwhile, beat the eggs and the sour cream together until smooth.

After the 10 minutes are up, pour the sour cream mixture over the blueberries. Bake an additional 40–45 minutes at 350 degrees.

12 servings.

Coffee Cake

¼ cup butter plus 1 t. for
   greasing pan
1 cup brown sugar
2 eggs, beaten
½ cup low-fat milk
1 T. lemon juice
2 cups wheat flour, sifted
   twice

1 t. baking powder
1 t. baking soda
1 t. vanilla
1 t. almond flavoring
¼ cup raisins
Cinnamon

Take 2 T. of the brown sugar and set aside. Grease a 9-inch cake pan with the 1 t. butter. Combine lemon juice and milk. Let stand. (Or use ½ cup sour milk instead of this mixture.) Sift flour, baking powder, and baking soda together. Cream butter and sugar. Add eggs and flavorings, beating well. Add alternately small amounts of flour and milk mixtures, beating well after each addition. Pour half of the batter in the pan. Sprinkle cinnamon, raisins, and reserved brown sugar over this. Add remainder of batter. Bake at 350 degrees for about 30 minutes.

Serves 12.

Coffee-Rum Cheese Pie

Crust:

4 zwieback, crushed   1 T. butter, melted

Combine and press onto bottom of 9-inch pie tin. Bake at 350 degrees for 3 minutes. Let cool.

Filling:

16 oz. ricotta cheese
½ cup brown sugar, packed
1 t. vanilla
1 t. coffee powder or granules

1 t. rum
1 T. flour
2 eggs, beaten (3 if they are
   small)

Combine ricotta, brown sugar, vanilla, and rum. Sprinkle coffee powder and flour over eggs, and beat well. Combine both mixtures. Pour over crust and bake at 350 degrees for 45–50 minutes.

Serves 12.

Gingerbread

¼ cup butter	¼ cup raisins
½ cup brown sugar	1 t. ginger
½ cup molasses	2 eggs, beaten until foamy
1½ cups wheat flour, sifted twice	½ t. baking soda
	½ cup low-fat milk

Cream butter. Add sugar, and cream again. Add molasses, raisins, ginger, and 1 cup flour. Mix in. Add remainder of flour, eggs, and soda warmed in milk. Mix again. Line 8 × 8-inch oiled pan with foil, which you then lightly oil. Dust with flour and shake out excess.

Pour gingerbread batter into pan and bake about 50 minutes in 325-degree oven. This is best if wrapped and chilled 3–6 days before serving.

16 servings.

Pumpkin Custard Pie

1 can (16 oz.) pumpkin, or 2 cups cooked pumpkin or winter squash, pureed	¼ t. nutmeg
	2 eggs, beaten
	½ cup low-fat milk
½ cup brown sugar	½ t. butter
1 t. cinnamon	1 T. molasses
¼ t. ginger	4 crushed zwieback

Preheat oven to 350 degrees. Butter 9-inch pie pan with ½ t. butter and dust with 1 T. crumbs.

Combine all ingredients. Pour into baking dish and bake for 30 minutes. Sprinkle remaining crumbs on top and bake for another 30 minutes. Chill before serving.

Serves 8.

Raspberry (or Peach) Kuchen

This is a variation of the blueberry kuchen, using half and half instead of sour cream. It is decidedly different in taste.

16 pieces zwieback	¾ cup brown sugar
1 quart raspberries (or any other berry or fruit. Try substituting 6 sliced peaches instead)	1 t. cinnamon
	2 eggs
	1 cup half and half

Crush zwieback and pour into bottom of 9 × 9-inch square pan. Sprinkle with half the cinnamon, and layer the fruit on top of this. Then top with the brown sugar, and bake for 10 minutes in a 400-degree oven.

Beat the eggs and half and half together. After the 10 minutes is up, pour the dairy mixture on top of the fruit, and bake at 350 degrees for 40–45 minutes more.

Serves 12.

Stovetop Apples and Raisins

1 large apple per person, cut into chunks	Cinnamon to taste (Optional: for a thicker sauce, add a little cornstarch)
1 T. water per person	
1 T. raisins per person	
Lemon juice to taste	

Place ingredients in a pot on low heat, and cook gently until tender. This is great served warm, and surprisingly sweet with absolutely no sugar.

Bread

My son and daughter are the bread makers in the family. They each take over the kitchen about once a week and turn out a batch that, unfortunately, does not keep us in full supply. There is nothing quite like good homemade bread, and these are soon gone—which means that we have to keep a supply of commercial breads in our freezer (see below).

David's Bread is a hearty, grainy, "old country"-style loaf. It's rich and somewhat sweet, which makes it an excellent snack, eaten without anything at all on it, with a glass of milk or cup of coffee.

Terri's Favorite Bread provides a healthy compromise recipe

that suits the taste for a softer-textured loaf preferred by many people. It's rich in protein because of the soy and wheat flour mixture.

Do *not* follow my son's suggestion unless you are the sort of person who can easily eat one salted peanut and stop. Stay out of the kitchen when these loaves come out of the oven!

David's Bread
(three loaves)

(As written for me after considerable coaxing.)
Start:

3 packets dry yeast in
2 cups warm water, with
1⅓ T. white sugar

Add water to the ingredients and stir well.
While the yeast is starting, mix in a large bowl or pot:

2 cups warm water	⅓ cup oil
2 cups white sugar	1⅓ T. salt

The water can be heated to facilitate thorough dissolution of the dry ingredients, but make sure it cools to below 110° or 115°F. before adding the yeast solution.

If you scurry through this, you'll have time to *butter* three loaf pans before the yeast foams all over the counter. Butter, as opposed to oil in the loaf pans, makes for easy removal of the loaves once cooked. Only a little is necessary. Don't forget the top edges.

Mix yeast with other solution and add about 3 pounds of whole-wheat flour. Mix well and dump onto kneading surface in the midst of more flour (this recipe takes about 4 pounds of flour for three loaves). Divide into thirds and knead thoroughly. Place in loaf pans and allow to rise in warm oven for an hour. The dough should double in size. Sometimes it has taken longer than an hour for the dough to rise, but I think this was due to difficulty in getting the oven to just the right temperature. It must be hot enough to make the yeast operate in a thick medium, but not so hot as to kill the yeast.

After the dough has risen sufficiently, bake 45 minutes at 350 degrees.

"After the loaves have cooled a little, try a slice while it is still hot enough to melt some butter."

(David is 6 feet 1 inch tall and has never weighed over 150 pounds in his entire life!)

Terri's Favorite Bread

Requires no kneading (two small loaves)

1 package yeast	1 T. sugar
1 cup warm water	2 t. salt
2½ cups white flour	½ cup warm water
½ cup soy flour	Butter
1 cup whole-wheat flour	

Put yeast in 1 cup warm water. Let stand while combining flours, sugar, and salt in bowl. Stir yeast to make sure it is dissolved, and add to flour mixture. Add the other ½ cup of water and mix to form a moist dough. Cover and let rise in a warm place until doubled.

Punch down and divide dough in two. Form into loaves and place into two buttered loaf pans. Let rise again until doubled. Bake in preheated oven at 375 degrees for 35 to 40 minutes, or until browned on top.

These loaves will have a hard crust yet will be very light inside.

Commercial Breads

I like whole-grain breads and my favorite commercial products are Pepperidge Farm and Earth Grains. However, these may not be available in all sections of the country. So, examine labels and, if you prefer whole grains, choose only those that clearly indicate "100 percent whole wheat." A label that reads "made with" 100 percent whole wheat usually means that the wheat has been blended with other flours.

However, you don't need to be a stickler. Many of the blended flours make excellent and nutritious loaves. And bread that has milk or eggs in the recipe will be relatively rich in protein. So, if you like the "Honey Bran" and "Wheat Berries" style of bread, you should feel free to use them. You are eating a very healthful diet when you follow the 28-Day Nutrition Plan and whether or not you always have whole-grain bread won't make a great deal of difference. The main difference in the end is fiber count—the white breads will have about 1 gram per slice, whereas the whole grains have about 3.

Miscellaneous

French Toast

2 slices whole-wheat bread   ¼ t. cinnamon
1 egg   ½ t. butter
1 T. skim milk

Beat egg and milk with cinnamon. Dip bread in egg mixture, coating both sides. Melt butter in a saucepan, and fry the bread, turning once, until golden brown on both sides.
Serves 1.

Cheese Toast

2 slices whole wheat bread   (Optional: 2 slices tomato)
1 oz. cheese, sliced thin

Place bread on foil on baking sheet. Arrange cheese, and tomato if desired, on bread, and place under broiler for a few minutes, until cheese is melted.
Serves 1.

Basic Pancake Mix

4 cups whole-wheat flour   1 t. salt
3 cups white flour   1 cup instant low-fat dry milk
1½ cups soy flour   ⅓ cup baking powder
2 cups wheat germ

To make pancakes, combine:

1½ cups mix   1 cup skim milk or water
2 eggs, beaten well   1 T. oil

Fry the pancakes in a very lightly oiled frying pan on medium heat.
Serving size: 2 medium.
Serves 4–6.

Herb Salt

Combine ¼ teaspoon of the following:

Thyme	Dried parsley
Dill weed	Salt
Celery seed	

Add ½ teaspoon basil

Combine ingredients and grind with a mortar and pestle. Store in a small herb jar. You can experiment with your own combinations. Herb salts are rich in flavor, and you will use less salt this way.

PART **III**

Your Fat-Burning Insurance Policy

16

BURNING FAT WHEN YOU THINK YOU CAN'T

For years I have been watching people buy exercise bicycles, barbells, rowing machines, and countless pieces of other home exercise equipment only to put them away in their closets and attics in short order. Then, in the fall of 1982, I discovered a marvelous little device that provides more weight-control insurance than any other piece of exercise equipment I have ever come across.

You can walk on it, dance on it, jog on it, or run on it; you can jump, bounce, and kick on it, and do calisthenics and strength training routines all at the same time if you choose to.

It's fun, it has tremendous calorie-burning payoff, it is used in the privacy of your own home, and it's available day or night, year-round, no matter what the weather.

It's called a minitrampoline or rebounder, and can be bought for as little as forty to fifty dollars at discount merchandise centers. More people from the Vanderbilt program continue to use this piece of equipment after buying it than have ever continued with exercise bicycles simply because it is so much more interesting and fun to use. Even if walking, jogging, or some active sport places highest in your preference, a rebounding routine affords an excellent fallback activity program when there is a tornado watch in the neighborhood, or the snow is 6 feet high, or you are short on time. It is a very worthwhile investment.*

In case you haven't as yet seen a "mini," they are made of strong

---

*The name "rebounder" is really a trade name, but it is used so commonly as to have become a generic term for the minitrampoline.

webbing attached to either a circular or a rectangular tubular steel frame 36 to 40 inches in diameter. The attachment is made by means of a network of springs that fit securely into the webbing and onto the frame. The frame is attached to legs that elevate it about 7 to 9 inches above the floor so that you can bounce on it. The legs are usually removable, which makes the mini semiportable. Most minis are tested to accommodate safely persons weighing up to 350 pounds.*

I am very enthusiastic about the weight-control benefits you can obtain by using this device. The routine that I am going to spell out for you will give you the same metabolic improvement benefits as brisk walking or even jogging. It is safe for overweight people who are otherwise in good health, but, naturally, if you suffer from any illness that requires medical supervision, you should check with your physician before using a rebounder.

Prior to beginning, however, I need to put rebounding in its proper perspective. On the one hand, many outlandish claims have been made for it by manufacturers and book writers selling re-bounding exercise programs; on the other hand, some traditional exercise physiologists have failed to appreciate its potential.

Enthusiasts like to claim that you burn more calories on a re-bounder than in walking or even running. The truth of the matter is that you may or may not! It all depends on your level of effort—so I will show you how to determine your own calorie expenditure in relation to walking or jogging.

Critics like to point out that, because of the rebound action of the minitrampoline, you get an assist in your movement and cannot acquire the same level of cardiovascular fitness as you can with brisk walking or jogging. Again, the truth of the matter is that you may or may not. It all depends upon whether you follow the principles I will now lay out for you.

---

*Before you purchase your mini, turn it upside down and examine it to be sure it has strong stitching and sturdy material where the springs are attached. Take off your shoes and give it a few test bounces. It should not feel significantly more flexible when you bounce with both feet together in the middle than it does when you place your feet a few inches apart. A great deal of flexibility in the center seems to tire the calves more quickly and, in some persons, it results in temporary soreness of the ankle joints until they get used to it.

Calorie Burning and Rebounder Fitness Principles

Any continuous whole-body movement done at Metabolic Breakthrough Intensity will burn approximately the same number of calories and yield the same cardiovascular improvement as any other continuous whole-body movement.

To determine whether you are burning the same number of calories and obtaining equivalent cardiovascular improvement in different activities, you can use either:

1. The method of perceived exertion, which is just a fancy way to say "going by your feelings," or

2. More exactly, you can use your heart rate and bring it up to the same level in the different activities.

Both methods are easy to use.

Gauging by Feeling

Assuming that you have become accustomed to the device, when you bounce on the minitrampoline at an intensity that feels equivalent in effort to walking at 3 MPH, you will be burning approximately the same number of calories as in walking. That is, the average person weighing about 154 pounds will be burning about 22 calories every 5 minutes. (Lighter persons will burn a little less, heavier persons a little more.)

When you bounce at an intensity that feels equivalent to walking briskly, for example, about 4 MPH, you will be burning about 33 calories every 5 minutes.

Table 16-1 presents a comparison of walking, rebounding, and running. You can see that running in place on the rebounder, with high knee lifts or kicks, is about equivalent to running at a pace of a mile in 9 minutes. It burns about 68 calories every 5 minutes.

Because of the assist given to your movement by the trampoline, you must move at a quicker pace than you would have to use if you propelled your body forward on a hard surface in order to experience equivalent effort.

Using Your Heart Rate as Your Guide

If you wish to improve the precision of your estimates of calorie burning in different activities, your heart rate furnishes a convenient and fairly reliable guide:

TABLE 16-1

Energy Expenditure in Walking, Rebounding, and Running

	MINUTES OF ACTIVITY					
ACTIVITY	5	10	15	30	45	60
Walking						
moderately, 3 miles per hour	22	44	66	132	198	264
briskly, 4 miles per hour	33	66	99	198	297	396
Rebounding						
brisk walking tempo,						
little foot lift	22	44	66	132	198	264
jogging tempo,						
4 to 6 inches of foot lift	33	66	99	198	297	396
running, high knee						
lifts, or kicks	68	136	204	408	612	816
Running (flat surface)						
a mile in 11½ minutes	47	94	141	282	423	564
a mile in 9 minutes	68	136	204	408	612	816
a mile in 8 minutes	73	146	219	436	655	874
a mile in 7 minutes	81	162	243	486	729	972
a mile in 6 minutes	88	176	264	528	792	1056
a mile in 5½ minutes	101	202	303	606	909	1212

1. Go for a walk at 3 MPH.* Take your pulse about 10 minutes into your walk. When you get your pulse up to a similar level in any other whole-body activity that you have become accustomed to, you will be burning approximately the same number of calories as in walking at that speed. That's about three times the number of calories that you would use sitting still (or about 22 every 5 minutes).

2. Go for a walk at 4 MPH. Repeat the process stated above. That pulse rate represents a caloric expenditure of a little over 4.5 times the number of calories it takes to sit still (or about 33 every 5 minutes).

3. If you can shuffle along at a slow jog, say at a mile in 11.5 minutes, try that and take your pulse once again. At that pulse

*Directions for determining your speed of walking are given on page 62.

rate you are burning calories between 6 and 6.5 times your sitting rate, or about 47 every 5 minutes.*

Reaching Metabolic Breakthrough Intensity on the Rebounder

Just as in walking or jogging, when you get your heart rate up into the 70 to 90 percent of maximum range you obtain a significant improvement in your cardiovascular condition. From a weight control standpoint, you reach metabolism improvement intensity because of the prolonged calorie-burning benefits you obtain following 30 minutes of activity.

Using your perceived effort as a guide, you reach Metabolic Breakthrough Intensity with brisk movement—anything that elevates your breathing to a noticeable degree, but not so high that you cannot continue to talk, whistle, or hum! You can be sure that you are obtaining metabolic improvement benefits when you reach the highest level of exertion that you can comfortably maintain for 30 to 45 minutes without ending up exhausted. Intensities greater than that are necessary if you want to become an Olympic star, but they are not necessary for weight control. You should end up feeling refreshed and eager for more the following day.

The cardiovascular conditioning you obtain on the rebounder is equal to that obtained with any other whole-body movement done at an equivalent heart rate. However, I must warn you that, if you use *only* the rebounder for physical activity, a treadmill or bicycle test of your cardiovascular condition will not yield an accurate estimate of your fitness. That is because exercise effects tend to be rather specific. If you bounce, your bouncing muscles and the vascular network that supplies them with oxygen will get into great shape; if you run, your running muscles and their blood supply networks develop. If you take a fitness test on equipment that requires good walking or running muscle development, and you have been doing some other exercise such as swimming, bouncing, or bicycling, the

*The methods I suggest afford a good approximation provided a person is equally proficient in each activity being compared. If you jog several miles a day but are an infrequent and lousy swimmer, your heart rate in the swimming pool will go up far beyond the level it would reach at a similar level of caloric expenditure in running. Although your heart is in good shape, the vascular network and muscle system involved in swimming are not. Therefore, you cannot use oxygen as efficiently as you do in running and the heart has to beat faster.

results of the test may be interpreted to mean that your heart is not in as good shape as it really is. The problem lies in the fact that you are being tested in an unaccustomed activity for which you have not become totally conditioned.

The Metabolic Breakthrough Rebounding Program

The Metabolic Breakthrough Rebounding Program has been used by persons up to 125 pounds over desirable weight. It is safe done as directed. By using your feelings or heart rate as a guide, it will give you the same weight-control benefits as walking, jogging, bicycling, or swimming.

If you have never bounced on a minitrampoline before, START SLOWLY AND FEEL YOUR WAY. Bouncing requires certain joints and muscles to contract and stretch in ways that are completely different from all other exercises. Although such reactions are rare, your ankle joints and calf muscles may experience some soreness the first few days because of the springlike action of the trampoline.

Start with 5 minutes of the warm-up exercises the first day that you use your rebounder—and that is all. Add more of the exercises and increase the duration of activity to gradually meet your weekly goal in the 28-Day Program.

Although the rebounder can be used as your sole source of metabolic improvement activity, most people like to mix up some bouncing with other activities. The greater the variety, the better your overall condition and the greater your enjoyment of your physical skills.

When using the rebounder, pay attention to:

posture and balance,
rhythm,
breathing, and
pace.

To *balance* correctly, stand in the center of the mat with feet slightly apart. (Always bounce barefoot or in stocking feet to avoid tearing up the webbing.)

For correct *posture,* keep your knees slightly bent and eyes looking straight forward. Let your hands hang comfortably, slightly in front of your waist.

Begin all exercises *slowly* and *rhythmically*. As soon as you become accustomed to the action of the trampoline, you will find that it is fun to bounce to music. Use any music that you enjoy dancing to or exercising with, and bounce with the beat.

Breath easily and deeply. After you have finished the short warm-up routine, begin to pace yourself at the intensity that you could continue for a full 30 to 45 minutes (whether or not you plan to go that long is not the issue—this is your guide to the appropriate intensity for shorter activity sessions as well as for the longer ones). If you get going too fast and begin to tire or get out of breath, return to one of the warm-up bounces until you recover.

Some suggested amounts of time for each exercise are in parentheses, but these are guidelines, not hard and fast rules. Practice the bounces until you can make transitions between them without losing a beat. You may find that your balance and coordination in a number of other activities will improve as a result of rebounding in this manner.*

Warm-up Routine

Spend 2 to 5 minutes doing the following warm-ups. Your effort should not exceed that of walking at a moderate pace.

1. Walking Warm-up: Stand in basic mat position. Keep the balls of your feet in constant contact with the mat and begin to lift first one heel and then the other in a slow rhythmic motion. Let the bounce occur naturally as the heels return to the mat. (1 minute)

2. Warm-up Bounce: Stand in basic mat position. Keeping the balls of your feet in constant contact with the mat, lift both heels simultaneously and return to the mat in slow rhythmic motion. The bounce will begin naturally. (1 minute)

---

*Almost all of the rebounder exercises can be done jogging or hopping in one place on the floor or rug. You do not need a rebounder to include them in your daily routine. However, it is much more fun to do them on a rebounder, and the wear and tear on your lower body joints is likely to be less if you like to do exercises of this kind on a frequent or daily basis.

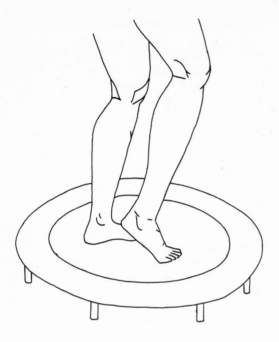

Exercise 1. Walking Warm-Up: the heel lift.

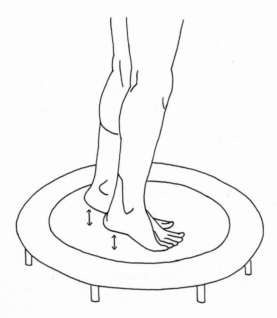

Exercise 2. Warm-Up Bounce: lift both heels and return.

3. Basic Bounce I: Standing in the center of the mat, keeping knees slightly bent, begin a slow rhythmic downward thrust with both feet. Keep your feet flat on the mat and in continual contact. Push down with your whole foot, or add an extra thrust with the balls of your feet, whichever feels most natural to you. (1 minute)

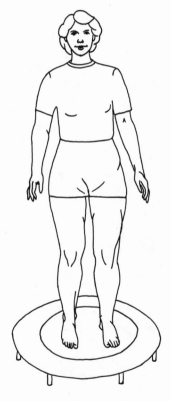

Exercise 3. Basic Bounce I: push down in a rhythmic motion. Feet do not leave the mat.

218 / Your Fat-Burning Insurance Policy

4. Arm Swings: This excellent exercise accomplishes two things at once. It conditions your arm and chest muscles as it begins to elevate your heart rate in preparation for the main series of rebounder exercises. Continuing with Basic Bounce I, extend your arms to the side and begin to rotate them from the shoulders. Coordinate two bounces to each rotation. Do 30 rotations in one direction, then reverse. This is also an excellent exercise for coordination: after completing 60 rotations with the Basic Bounce, make transitions to the Walking Warm-up and to the Warm-up Bounce, continuing to swing your arms without losing a beat. (2 minutes)

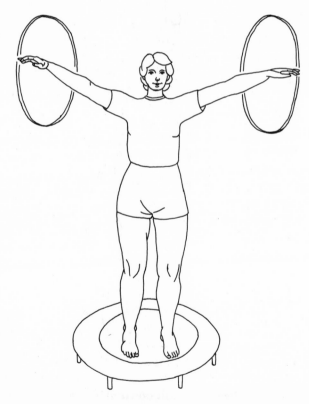

Exercise 4. Arm Swings: rotate your arms as you bounce.

Metabolic Breakthrough Routine

5. *Mini-jog:* Using Warm-up Walk motion, lifting first one heel and then the other, speed up the tempo to a brisk pace. Your feet never leave the mat. Swing your arms vigorously in the motion they would naturally follow in a brisk walk. (2 minutes)

6. *Basic Bounce II:* This is a higher level of intensity applied to the Basic Bounce motion. Increase the speed of the Basic Bounce and almost reach the point where your feet are about to leave the mat at the height of your bounce. The deeper you thrust your feet down into the mat at the bottom of your bounce, the greater the

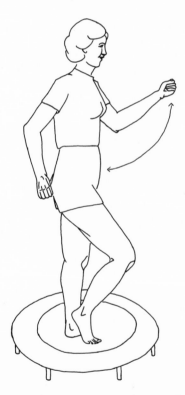

Exercise 5. Mini-jog: swing your arms vigorously; fast walking motion.

rebound effect and the higher you go at the top of the bounce (not illustrated). (2 minutes)

7. *Full Jog:* The Full Jog on the rebounder is simply an extension of the Walking Warm-up or Mini-jog motion. Keep your upper body relaxed and begin to lift your feet 4 to 6 inches off the mat with each step. When you begin to use this jogging motion, do not exceed the intensity of a brisk walk for the first few days. (2 minutes)

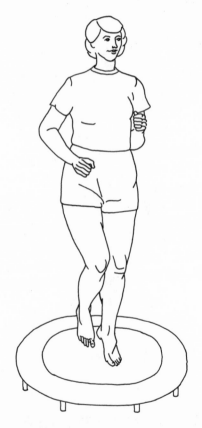

Exercise 7. Full Jog: lift your feet 4 to 6 inches off the mat.

8. Basic Bounce III: Basic Bounce III is what people usually associate with the rebounder. Deepen the thrust you have been using at Level II until your feet begin to leave the mat. Start with a bounce that takes you 1 inch into the air and see how it feels. You will bounce higher and easier if you raise your hands just slightly, and with palms facing down, combine a gentle downward thrust

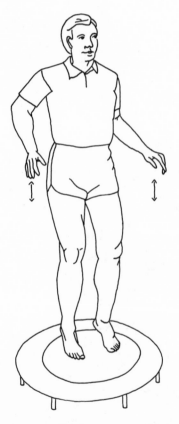

Exercise 8. Basic Bounce III: bounce as high as is comfortable, adding downward motions with hands.

with your hands and arms each time you land on the mat. Do not exceed the intensity of a brisk walk for the first few days. (2 minutes)

9. Forward Kick: As soon as you feel comfortable with the previous exercises, you will be ready for some that require a bit more coordination and effort. The Forward Kick is done to a "one count" or a "two count." In the one-count version, just lift your right foot

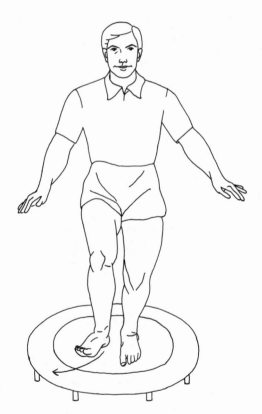

Exercise 9. Forward Kick: alternate legs, kicking forward about 4 inches.

about 4 inches off the mat and kick forward. Bring it back to the mat as you simultaneously kick forward with the left. The bounce takes care of itself. In the two-count version, which requires more effort, you add an extra bounce to the kick. While the right foot is extended, you intentionally bounce again on the left. Return the right foot as you kick forward with the left, and add a bounce on the right foot. Thus, it's two beats to a kick. (2 minutes)

10. Side Kick: Same as the Forward Kick, except that you kick out to the side rather than straight ahead. (2 minutes)

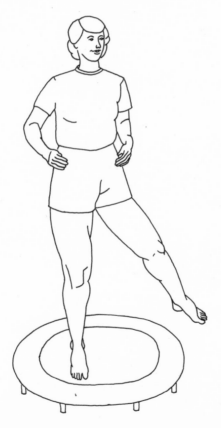

Exercise 10. Side Kick: kick out to the side, alternating legs.

11. Double Shuffle: Stand in basic position with weight on the balls of your feet. Slide one foot forward and the other back. Then reverse: slide front foot back, and back foot forward. Feet do not leave the mat. Think light and it gets easy! When you master the motion, turn your whole body 45 degrees to the right in the middle of a shuffle step without losing a beat. Complete two or more shuffle steps in that direction, and return to center. Then rotate left 45 degrees. Practice will improve your timing and coordination. (2 minutes)

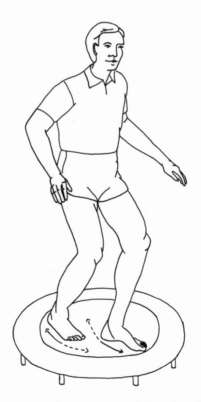

Exercise 11. Double Shuffle: alternate sliding feet forward and back. Feet do not leave the mat.

12. *Skip Rope:* No, not with a real rope. This is an invisible-rope skip. Imagine you have a rope in your hands and begin a rhythmic swing, stepping or jumping in your preferred rope-skipping motion. (2 minutes)

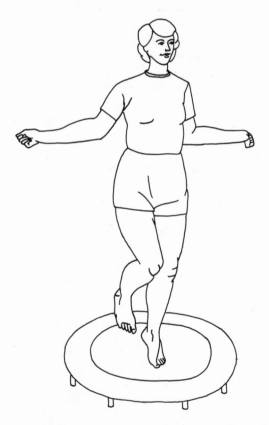

Exercise 12. Skip Rope: use an imaginary rope in a skipping motion.

Upper Body Conditioning on the Minitrampoline

The following series of exercises will give you the same upper-body conditioning that you obtain from a calisthenic routine with a couple of added metabolism improvement benefits: because you are doing them on a rebounder, you are burning at least twice the number of calories you would otherwise. As your coordination improves, you can do them with increasing vigor. When you include them in your full 30 minutes of rebounder activity, you will continue to burn extra calories for hours after you finish.

13. Breaking Chains: While continuing in the Mini-jog or Basic Bounce motion, make fists with both hands and bring them up in front of your chest about 6 inches apart *(a)*. Raise your elbows so that your bent arms are parallel to the floor. Imagine that you are gripping a chain. Break it by thrusting your elbows backward *(b)*, and then, in a separate motion, fling your arms to the side as though you were throwing the pieces away *(c)*. Keep repeating the set of motions. Establish a rhythm to go with your bounce. Two beats to each arm motion seems to work best. (1 minute)

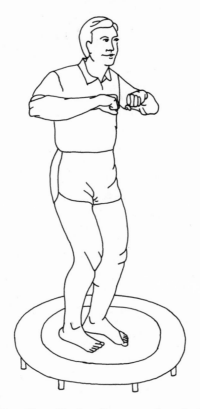

Exercise 13a. Breaking Chains: fists together in front of chest.

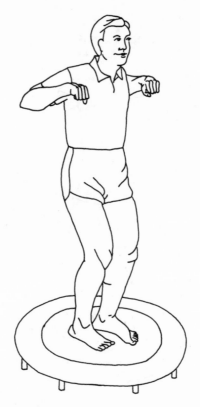

Exercise 13b. Breaking Chains: thrust elbows back and break the chain.

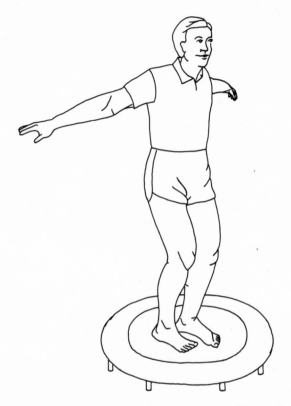

Exercise 13c. Breaking Chains: fling arms to side and throw the pieces away.

14. Reach for the Stars: This one offers exceptional conditioning for your shoulders and upper body. Continuing with either the Mini-jog or Basic Bounce, bring your hands up to shoulder level. Thrust upward, high over your head, to grab some stars, and then return your hands to shoulder level. Coordinate your upward thrusts with your bounce, using either a one or a two count with each thrust. (1 minute)

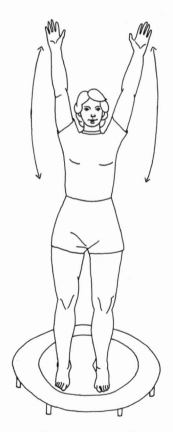

Exercise 14. Reach for the Stars: coordinate upward thrusts with your bounce.

15. Biceps Bounce: Continuing with Mini-jog or Basic Bounce motion, imagine that you have a dumbbell in each hand, tense your biceps, and do arm (biceps) curls. You can use light weights (3 to 6 pounds) or a book in each hand if you choose. Do one or two bounces to each arm motion. (1 minute)

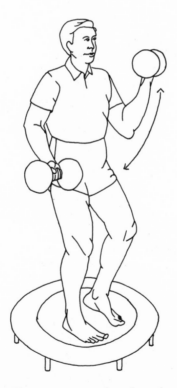

Exercise 15. Biceps Bounce: use real or imaginary dumbbells and do arm curls as you bounce.

16. Karate Punch: This is just one of many karate moves you can make while bouncing. Continue with a slow jog or bounce motion. Bring one hand to the waist, and punch vigorously forward with the other at solar plexus (pit of the stomach) height. Alternate bringing one hand back to the waist, and punching with the other straight forward. In authentic form, the fist that is brought to the waist is rotated palm side up, while the fist in the forward punch is rotated palm side down. This exercise is excellent for coordination and will require a bit of practice. Use either a one- or two-count bounce to

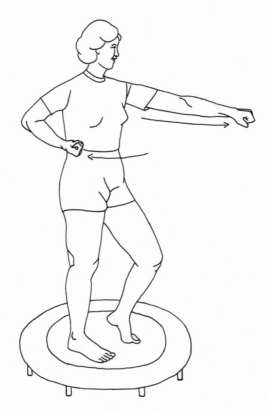

Exercise 16. Karate Punch: alternate straight forward punches and returning fists to waist.

each punch and, if you punch vigorously, you will be surprised at the workout you will get. (1 minute)

17. Jumping Jacks: Make a transition from the Basic Bounce to a straddle hop, that is, jump and land with both feet a few inches out to the side. Be careful not to jump so wide that you hit the edge of the rebounder webbing. When the rhythm is established, swing your arms out to the side and up over your head, using one or two bounces at the top and bottom of the arm movement. This is another vigorous exercise that's good for your coordination. (1 minute)

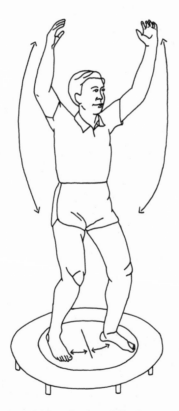

Exercise 17. Jumping Jacks: do straddle hops a few inches to the side as you swing your arms up over your head.

18. Atlas Special I: This exercise is one example of how you can use your time on the mini for honest-to-goodness strength training and toning exercises. Continue with a comfortable slow bounce or Mini-jog, make a fist with your right hand, and turn it palm side up. Grab the wrist with your left hand and try to lift the right as you apply opposing force with your left *(a)*. Gradually let your right hand rise against the pressure of the left, and then let the left hand

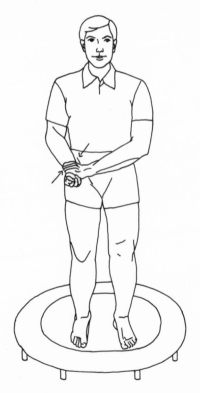

Exercise 18a. Atlas Special I: apply continual pressure as the wrist forces the hand upward.

force it back down as the right resists all the way *(b)*. Use a six-count up and a six-count down beat. Repeat three times, and then switch hand positions. Once you get comfortable with this exercise, investigate all the positions in which you can apply this principle as you bounce. You are building muscle tone and conditioning your upper body according to a time-tested principle of strength training. But, in addition, you are burning twice the calories that you would burn if you did these exercises standing still, and you are getting extra metabolism improvement benefits to boot. (2 minutes)

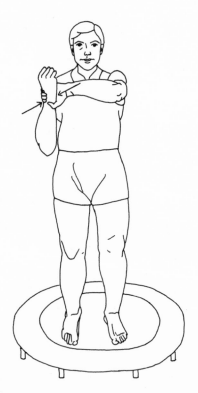

Exercise 18b. Atlas Special I: apply continual pressure as the hand forces the wrist down.

19. Atlas Special II: Clasp your hands in front of you, close to your body, chest high. Let your right hand push the left to the side, as the left resists all the way. Then reverse, pushing with the left, resisting with the right. About 6 bounces to each motion. (2 minutes)

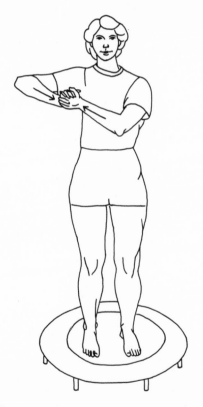

Exercise 19. Atlas Special II: Apply continual opposing pressure as one arm forces the other to the side, then reverse direction.

Repeat the exercises of your choice until you reach the daily time goal of your Metabolic Breakthrough Program. Be sure to cool down for at least 2 minutes with a slow jog or bounce before you step off the trampoline.

As soon as you become familiar with the various routines I have suggested, be inventive. Create your own bounces. As long as you keep the pace at Metabolic Breakthrough Intensity, you will be burning the same calories as in walking or jogging, and you will also be obtaining some important upper-body conditioning that you do not normally obtain in those activities.

17

THE BASIC EIGHT: STRETCHING EXERCISES FOR ACTIVE PEOPLE

This set of flexibility exercises is called the Basic Eight because it works the most important muscles and regions of the body for active people: calves, hamstrings (muscles at the rear of your legs), stomach, and lower back. If you already have an established stretching and toning program that does not contain exercises such as these, be sure to add them to it.

This is an intentionally brief stretching program—it is designed to be the perfect complement to the Metabolic Breakthrough Activity Program without asking you to devote more time than is absolutely necessary. While stretching exercises do not burn many calories, *they keep your body in shape to do the ones that do.*

The exercises take only 5 minutes to run through and you should do them a minimum of once a day. They will prevent soreness and injury, and, in fact, they are especially useful if you already suffer from aches in your legs or stiffness in your lower back.

If you are the kind of person who wakes up feeling very stiff in the morning, try doing them before going to bed at night, as well as in the morning. Done several times a day, they can completely relieve minor back problems. Of course, if you suffer from chronic back pain, you should check with your physician or physical therapist to be sure you are doing the correct set of exercises for your particular problem.

In all stretches, never push yourself to the point of pain. "Feel" the stretch, and stop there. In time, the distance or degree of your stretch will increase naturally.

1. Sit on the floor, legs crossed in "little tailor" position. Bend forward from the hips, keeping your back straight. Reach out as far forward as you can with your hands to touch the floor. Stretch your shoulder joints as well as your hips. Hold this position for 10 to 20 seconds and then relax.

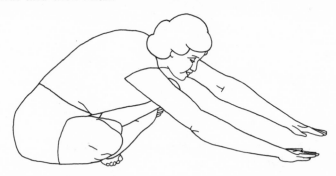

Exercise 1. Bend forward from the hips, keeping your back straight.

2. Straighten your legs out flat in front of you. Bend forward from the hips, point your toes back toward your head, and work toward grasping your toes with your fingertips (many persons can only reach to their ankles when they first try this exercise—if this is true of you, do not force yourself to go beyond the point of comfort; your flexibility will increase gradually). Hold the stretch for 10 to 20 seconds. This is good for the hip joints, calves, and hamstrings.

3. Lie flat on the floor, arms out to the side, legs together. Bending your right knee, place your right foot under your left knee. Keep your shoulders flat to the floor and rotate your lower body at the hips to the left. Try to touch the inside of your right knee to the floor on your left side. Turn your head to look to the right, out over your extended right arm. You can help your knee toward the floor with a little assist from your left hand, but do not force the stretch —you do not have to touch the floor to feel a good stretch. This exercise helps increase lower-back flexibility (and relieves existing stiffness). Hold about 10 seconds and reverse (left foot under right knee, etc.).

4. Lie flat on the floor, legs together. Bring your right knee to your chest (leg is bent) and, holding the knee with both hands, press

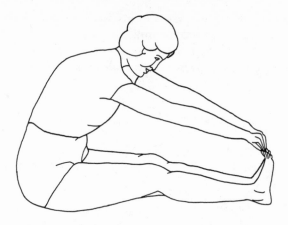

Exercise 2. Keep legs flat to the floor and bend forward from the hips; reach for your ankles if you can't reach your toes.

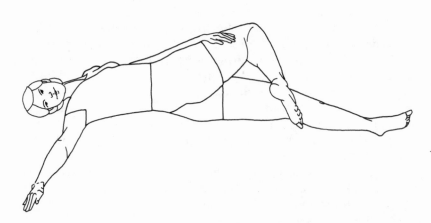

Exercise 3. Rotate from the hips; do not force the knee to the floor. Excellent for the lower back.,

it *gently* toward your chest. Head and shoulders can come up off the floor, if you like, or you can use a pillow under your head for this and the next three exercises. Hold it for 10 seconds and reverse legs. This is a lower-back exercise.

5. Bring both knees to your chest, gently press them closer with both hands, and hold for about 10 to 20 seconds. This is another excellent lower-back exercise.

6. From the position you are already in for Exercise 5, continue to hold on to your right knee while you grasp the big toe of your left foot with your left hand. Straighten the left leg out, up toward the ceiling, as far as you can, continuing to hang on to the big toe. Hold for at least 10 seconds and reverse. This works the calves, hamstrings, and lower back as a unit.

7. Place hands palms down under your buttocks. Bending at the

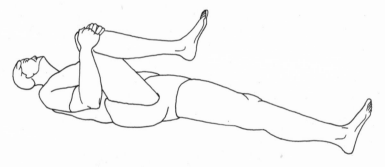

Exercise 4. Gently press the knee to the chest.

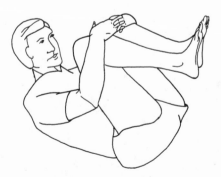

Exercise 5. Gently press both knees to the chest.

hips, bring your knees up halfway to your chest and do a bicycling motion for 10 seconds (or ten rotations) *(a)*. Then lower your legs straight out in front of you to within 6 inches of the floor and do flutter kicks for 10 seconds (or ten repetitions) *(b)*. Repeat bicycle

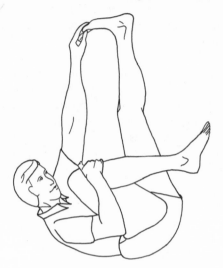

Exercise 6. Try to straighten the leg as far as possible.

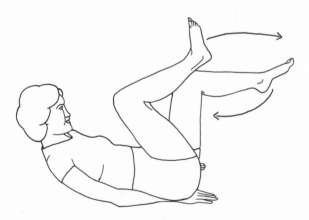

Exercise 7a. Bicycle motion: alternate with flutter kicks.

motion alternating with flutter kicks until you feel some strain in your stomach area. This is an excellent tummy toner and back exercise that takes the place of sit-ups. However, if you already suffer from chronic lower-back pain, do not do this exercise without getting your therapist's advice. Your problem may require another stomach muscle strengthener.

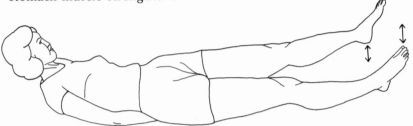

Exercise 7b. Flutter kicks: keep feet a few inches off the floor. Alternate with bicycle motion.

8. Finish up with a shoulder stand, legs extended up over your body in any way that is comfortable. If you cannot do a shoulder stand, simply place your legs up on a chair and relax for 30 seconds (see Alternate Exercise 8). This is good for your circulation, helps reduce swelling around the ankles, and will relieve "drawing pains" in the legs. If you experience pain in the extremities during the night, do this before going to bed. However, if you suffer from hypertension, do not do any exercise that requires you to lift your legs up over your head, as in a shoulder stand, without consulting your physician.

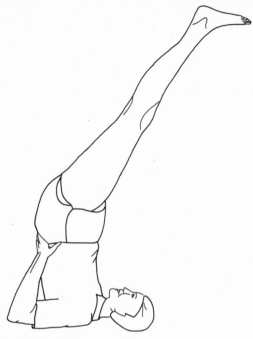

Exercise 8. Shoulder stand: excellent for the circulation.

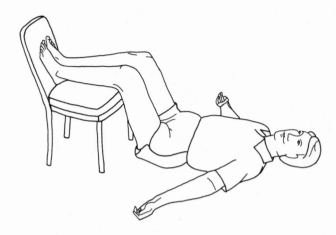

Alternate Exercise 8. A substitute for the shoulder stand. A relaxation posture, good for the circulation.

PART **IV**

The Scientific Background

A SHORT HISTORY OF OBESITY

Your eating preferences and your body weight are determined by many factors—biological, psychological, and social. The biological roots are deeply embedded in the history of the human race.[1]

Before we get into that history, take a few moments to answer the questions in the following Eating Habits Test. This test focuses on the psychological and environmental factors that most people associate with being overweight.

1. Do you tend to overeat at parties or other festive social occasions (such as holidays or weddings)?
2. Once you have started eating a favorite food, do you tend to have trouble stopping?
3. Do you tend to overeat on weekends?
4. Does the smell of food tend to make you hungry?
5. Do you sometimes eat when you are not really hungry?
6. Do you tend to eat at times when you are nervous, tense, or anxious?
7. Do you tend to eat at times when you are depressed, blue, or discouraged?
8. Do you tend to eat at times when you are angry or irritable?
9. Do you tend to overeat on foods that are particularly high in calories (the foods on my DC list, such as candy, desserts, anything sweet or high in fat, or both)?
10. If your favorite foods are in your home, do you end up eating them even when you are trying to cut calories or use some special diet?

If you have answered one or more of these questions, even all of them, in the "yes" direction, CONGRATULATIONS. You have passed the test. You have answered just like any perfectly normal human being!

I am not kidding you and I am not trying to be funny. I know that you have taken quizzes like this before, if not in a famous diet manual, then in one of the popular magazines that's introducing the diet of the month. If you answer "yes" to a certain number of questions, the writer leads you to believe you have some kind of "eating problem." You have what the experts call "maladaptive eating habits" or "problem foods."

And then what happens? You try the new miracle diet, and you try to employ the latest psychological gimmick, only to end up kicking yourself the moment you succumb to one of your favorite foods because it somehow pops up right in front of your nose and it tastes so good! You ask yourself, "Why have I failed?" and, because of all the nonsense that's been written about how easy it is to employ the newest tricks to control your eating, you attribute your failure to something emotional or psychological. You must be abnormal because, instead of relaxing or meditating as you were supposed to do, you have eaten in response to some emotion. And if you plead "circumstances," such as a party or other celebration instead of your emotional state, you have an immoral, despicable, and shameful lack of willpower!

I want to tell you right off, drawing upon my experience as a psychologist, that in the vast majority of instances—perhaps 95 percent of the 2,000 or so persons that have come through the Vanderbilt program—there is nothing at all wrong with people, mentally, morally, emotionally, or spiritually, that causes them to be overweight. Given the circumstances that I am about to discuss, it's perfectly natural.

It's natural because there are some very powerful, underlying biological forces that influence your eating preferences and your weight. These forces interact with the nature of your particular environment, and together these biological and environmental forces have a very subtle influence on your thoughts and emotions. You may not be aware of the process. When you become aware of how this works you will see that there is no need for any guilt, blame, or shame in connection with your eating habits or your weight. And you will also see that there is nothing wrong with you, either.

You will be rid of any emotional or psychological burden that you have mistakenly associated with your weight problem when you understand the answers to the following questions:

1. Why does the human body store fat in the first place?

2. Why do women store more fat than men, and have a much harder time losing it?

3. Why do you, and virtually all omniverous mammals from rats to humans, have a preference for foods that have a great potential for increasing that fat storage—those DC foods that are sweet and high in fat content, or both?

When you have the answers to these questions, you will see why it is natural, under the present circumstances of life in the Western world, for the average American, you included, to be a good 20 pounds over his or her most desirable weight, and for perhaps 40 to 60 million of us to be more than 20 percent over desirable weight.

The Historical Perspective

When mankind first appeared as a distinct species several million years ago we faced a rather precarious existence. We were preyed on by other animals, were frequently felled by infectious disease at an early age, and were victims of a rather uncertain food supply. Even as recently as Roman times, the average life span was only about 30 years, owing both to a high rate of infant mortality and to disease.

Our bodies developed special capacities for survival through natural processes of adaptation and selection. For the most part, we were hunter/gatherers. In general, the males did the hunting and developed both the physical endurance and the mental-planning ability to run down deer and corner mountain lions. A relatively large muscle mass together with relatively little body fat was an advantage. In all likelihood, after a kill far from home, the males simply ate until their hunger was satisfied, rested, and then brought the remains back to whereever the females and children were encamped. Chances are that females may have endured more frequent and longer periods of life in negative caloric balance during food shortages than did males.

Females contributed to the gathering of food that grew naturally in the environment and had primary responsibility for the care and nourishment of the young. Since, as I mentioned earlier, it takes between 40,000 and 80,000 extra calories to carry a fetus to term, and about 850 extra calories to nurse the infant each day, it was to an evolutionary advantage that females add relatively more fat to their bodies than males. In case of a food shortage, 15 extra pounds of fat contain enough energy to keep a baby alive for about three or four months.

Evolutionary pressures favoring the survival of a relatively fat lineage probably increased as more of the human race turned to agriculture and away from hunting and gathering. Up until the development of modern agricultural techniques in the Western world, rather than increasing the dependability of the food supply, a reliance on cultivated crops has only resulted in more severe famines when a primary crop fails because of weather, insects, or blight. The severe famine in Africa in the spring and summer of 1983 illustrates this point: thousands of people died and millions more will experience lifelong aftereffects of severe malnutrition.

The storage of fat on the human body is actually an extremely convenient and efficient mechanism for coping with such circumstances and providing long-term energy. It's concentrated energy, in comparison with carbohydrate or protein. Even when there is an abundance of food, humans metabolize energy continually, but eat intermittently. When food is short, we may have to go many months taking in less energy than we need to expend in order to maintain bodily processes and any other activity necessary to our existence. It was an evolutionary advantage to develop a concentrated form of energy storage. Not only does fat contain 9 calories of metabolizable energy per gram, in comparison with carbohydrate or protein, which have about 4, but the form of storage is extremely efficient. Because of the way fat cells are constituted, with about 70 to 80 percent fat, and only 20 to 30 percent water and other cellular materials, we can concentrate about 3500 calories in each pound. If necessary, 40 pounds of fat could supply the fuel to walk about 1400 miles during a migration. And the body at rest can burn fat almost exclusively, which means that an extra 40 pounds of fat can supply resting energy needs for several months if food becomes very scarce.

If we had to store the energy contained in 40 pounds of fat in a carbohydrate-related form, as glycogen in our liver or muscle storage sites, it could add over 275 pounds to our bodies! That's because the storage of glycogen does not afford the same concentration of energy. In addition to containing only 4 calories per gram, each gram of glycogen requires 3 to 4 grams of water in solution. This means that we can only get about 500 calories worth of energy out of a pound of glycogen storage.

So, the concentrated storage of energy as fat was a nice solution to the problem of an uncertain food supply, and the ability to store somewhat more of it on the female an important factor in the survival of offspring. I suspect, too, that selective factors relating to the resistance to infectious disease also contributed to enhanced fat storage, since, during the fever that develops in response to infection, the metabolic rate goes up about 7 percent with each degree of temperature. A little extra fat provided energy to prolong life in the face of illness and was in reality an asset before the advent of modern public health practices and antibiotics. It seems a bit ironic that our ability to store a substantial amount of fat, which was an asset in previous times and helped people survive through their reproductive years, has now become a liability. Today, the major threats to longevity, at least in the Western world, have switched from infectious disease and famine in early life to degenerative diseases, frequently aggravated if not caused by obesity, later in life.

But what about that preference for sweet and fatty foods—the juicy steaks and fried chicken, the candy, cookies, cakes, and soft drinks?

That liking for sweetness, and for sweetness or saltiness in combination with high fat content, is built into your genes.

A preference, in fact a *drive,* to overindulge whenever such foods are, or *were,* available is part and parcel of our biological equipment for survival.

I say "when such foods are or *were* available" because it is only within the last 300 years that persons in the Western world—and only in the Western world—have had a dependable food supply. I mentioned earlier that over two-thirds of the human race still faces periodic famines. So did our own ancestors for millions of years—up until about 300 years ago for those of us with European ancestry. If you face an uncertain tomorrow, you better stock up today—which makes it a good idea from a survival standpoint to prefer the food characteristics that can lay down fat quickly in order to gain weight whenever the food supply is plentiful. Under the usual conditions of human existence, which still operate over much of the world, the weight you gain this year will only come off next in the process of supplying the energy you need in a time of shortage.

So our preference for food characteristics that lead to weight gain is perfectly natural. In fact, it is shared by almost all mammals that have faced frequent uncertainty in their food supply and that have developed the capacity to metabolize a wide variety of foods during the evolutionary process. Even rats will react to the free availability of the same kinds of foods that humans respond to and overeat on things like peanut butter, chocolate candy, salami, sweetened milk, etc., to the point of obesity.

The point I am trying to make for you is that it is *unnatural* to resist fattening foods when they are freely available in your environment.

There are at least two million years of evolutionary wisdom in our genes that virtually *dictate* eating behavior in response to foods that are sweet, fatty, or, especially, both. And variety in our food contributes to the turn-on. There is a large body of research with animals as well as humans to prove this. A measly few generations of plenty are simply not enough to have brought about changes in that overwhelming biological predisposition. And you should be thankful—if it had not been present in your family line, you might not be here today!

While the natural course of evolutionary events seemed to have created that preference for sweets and fat, we did not develop a discriminating mechanism for choosing the most wholesome sweetness or fats. And we have not developed a finely tuned "turn-off" mechanism to put an end to our eating behavior when we've had enough if our calories are put to us in an unnaturally concentrated form. Evidently, because of the general infrequency of continued plenty, a "turn-off" switch may not have been as important to our survival. Furthermore, concentrated, processed sweetness in abundance is a very recent phenomenon. It has only been for about 100 years that refined sugar has been affordable and in plentiful supply. Up until then, our sweetness came from unrefined sources that contained essential vitamins, minerals, and large amounts of fiber as well as calories. Considering the bulk that accompanies most unprocessed forms of sweetness, we really didn't need to have a sweetness turn-off; the bulk would take care of it. To illustrate this point, in terms of calories, it takes two whole grapefruits to equal one soft drink, or six fresh apples to equal one piece of pie. I am sure you can see the rationale for my AC/DC formula—it becomes very hard to stay fat when you return to the more natural way of eating, substituting natural sweetness for the concentrated, processed variety.

But food manufacturers work hard to please our appetites, and research in their laboratories has shown them how to capitalize on our natural predispositions. Sugar helps increase the attractiveness of bologna, and of peanut butter and catsup. A little bit of salt increases the palatability of chocolate chip cookies. I am not being critical with these observations—I am just demonstrating to you that your food preferences have a biological basis. Within each culture, enterprising individuals put their brains to work to dress up the foods that are available. They add just the right amounts of fat, sugar, and salt, blended with any other flavor that will mix well with them, and develop the most enticing (and salable) concoctions.

The point of this discussion is that, if you want to turn on an appetite anywhere in the world, you can capitalize on some combination of sweetness and fat, plus a little salt and other flavorings. And it's ridiculous to think that anyone, including you, should possess some sort of unnatural, superhuman willpower to override the pressures of our genetic heritage.

Indeed, as one of my colleagues remarked, when good, tasty food is available, *dieting* (not overeating!) is an eating disorder.

So the scene is set for overeating in the face of good and plenty, and for storing the fat to protect us against the impending shortage —except that the naturally occurring shortage never occurs. Instead of famines we have diets, which don't succeed in keeping our weight where we want it to be for very long, but do succeed in giving our fat-storing mechanisms the practice for which they were intended.

Unfortunately, those of us who feel the greatest pressure to lose weight in our culture—I'm referring to women—have a built-in protection against dieting that seems to exceed the defensive abilities of men. It's no secret that women lose weight more slowly than men in just about every weight-control program. The reasons are not all entirely clear, but they are related to initial differences in body weight and body composition, and to the hormone and enzyme structures that lead to an increased ability to store fat in the first place.

In general, being lighter, women do not need as many calories as men because total energy needs are closely tied to body weight. The heavier you are, the more fuel it takes to move yourself around. But, in addition, women do not need as many calories *per pound* of body weight to sustain basal metabolic processes. Men have a higher muscle to fat ratio in their bodies, and you will recall that muscle tissue burns more calories than fat tissue at rest. The metabolic cutback in response to dieting may also be more drastic in women than in men. Furthermore, because women cannot build muscle as easily as men, physical exercise may not facilitate the development of additional calorie-burning muscle tissue to quite the same extent that it does in men.

The cards do seem to be stacked against women when it comes to losing weight. Unfortunately, most popular diet programs just encourage women to diet harder than ever, and this is exactly the way to turn on their superior fat conservation powers. You're just knocking your head against a wall when you follow that kind of dietary advice. That "remedy" only increases the severity of the problem.

The key to successful weight control in conditions of plenty is to *stop dieting* and begin to *burn enough calories* to match your natural appetite.

Your fat-burning power is maximized when you follow the principles of the Metabolic Breakthrough Activity Program. In Chapter 21, I present an analysis of fifty-five physical training studies that proves the point and shows that the differences between men and women in response to physical activity may not be significant when you adhere to its principles.

19

THE GENETICS AND BIOCHEMISTRY OF OBESITY

It seems as though some of us were meant to be fatter than others.

In the preceding chapter, I discussed the reasons why human beings like the taste of foods that can easily add to our fat storage. I also outlined the evolutionary pressures that developed our ability to store fat, especially in the female.

I want to tell you now about the genetic and biochemical factors —those hormones and enzymes—that make it easier for *some* individuals to store *more* fat than others. These factors make it harder for such persons to lose weight. If you have had a persistent weight problem that has so far defied reasonable efforts to control it, you are likely to see yourself described here. With your new understanding, I hope you will find it easier to be patient with your body.

I also intend to show you how your eating and activity habits interact with your hereditary predisposition. You will see that it is really a fifty–fifty proposition.

Do you have a mother or father, or a close relative, who is overweight? When you look in the mirror, can you see a similar body build? Are you bulging in pretty much the same places as this forebear or relative? If so, you can be quite certain that some hereditary factor is operating in your own case to make it easier to gain weight.

But that disposition only sets the stage—you have tremendous power to influence the ultimate outcome. In Chapter 22 I will show you how people with varying degrees of genetic predispositions to obesity have nevertheless achieved permanent success using Metab-olism Breakthrough principles. And this, I hope, will fortify your own will to succeed.

Heredity and Obesity

I want to start with a discussion of the animal research because it is considerably easier to observe the role of heredity in the body weight of animals than it is in human beings. With animals, we can construct experiments that give us greater control over both genetic and environmental factors.

Working in the laboratory with rats and mice, which have physio-logical and metabolic processes remarkably similar to those of hu-mans, scientists have identified strains of naturally obese animals. Recent advances in genetics and biochemistry have helped to ex-plain the mechanisms that account for their differences from the naturally lean.

In some animals (e.g., the Zucker rats and *ob/ob* mice) a single gene abnormality triggers a network of central nervous system, hormone, and enzyme changes at a particular stage of these ani-mals' developments. They begin to overeat and become grossly obese. After a time, their weight begins to level out and they return to a near-normal level of food intake. However, even on a reduced intake, they continue to maintain their degree of overweight.[1]

If researchers restrict the food intake of these animals so that they cannot gain any more weight than animals that do not have the genetic defect, the animals still get fat. The power of the fat-storing hormones and enzymes (in particular, insulin and adipose tissue lipoprotein lipase) is so great that the lean tissue in their bodies is robbed of the nutrients needed for growth.

On the surface, these naturally fat but food-restricted animals don't look much different from the naturally lean. However, their bodies have four or five times as much fat. Their hearts, kidneys, and skeletal muscle systems are reduced up to half in size so that the fat mass can increase to exactly the same proportion of their body weight as if they had eaten freely.[2]

As the fat mass in some of these strains of animals grows larger and larger because of the increased activity of the fat-storing hor-mones and enzymes, the fat cells may lose sensitivity to other hormones (the catecholamines and growth hormone) that mobilize the fat for use as energy. These changes make it very easy to store fat, and very difficult to mobilize it for fuel.

Single gene defects like those found in the animals I have just described are probably extremely rare in humans. It is important to study these animals, however, because we discover just which hormones and enzymes express the defect. Then we can look for the less severe deviations from normal and see to what extent they influence our weight. This, in turn, allows us determine whether our eating and activity habits can change the levels of these hormones and enzymes and we can take corrective action.

In humans, as in most strains of animals that do not show a simple genetic defect, obesity seems to be influenced by a variety of constitutional and environmental factors. It's a combination of hereditary predispositions interacting on a fifty–fifty basis with eating and activity habits. Among different strains of animals, some fatten more easily than others the moment they are given extra calories in a tasty form.[3] Some strains may multiply fat cells as they gain weight while others get fat primarily by enlarging the cells they were born with.[1] Most strains will overeat and get fat on a diet that's high in fat and sugar. And, while most animals will lose weight when they are returned to a standard laboratory chow diet (low in fat, high in carbohydrate and protein), at least one normally lean strain does not. And we have just demonstrated in our research at Vanderbilt that a naturally slim strain, fattened on a high-fat diet, can be made resistant to weight loss by repeated fasting.

Because the animals used in research have metabolic processes similar to those of humans, the variability across different strains is very similar to the variability among human beings. Just as in the animal models, some humans appear to have genetic factors that operate so strongly to conserve energy and shunt calories off to their fat cells that they seem to get fat on any but the most Spartan of diets. Others just have a tendency toward obesity. Some humans lose weight easily every time they diet, and gain it back just as easily (and then some) if they ever return to eating foods high in fat and sugar. In contrast, other humans find that it gets harder and harder to lose weight each time they try a new diet. And then there is the opposite extreme of hard-to-fatten humans. These folks can eat anything. Their bodies seem capable of burning an unlimited num-

ber of calories and storing no more than the bare minimum necessary to support and cushion their internal organs.

It is easy to create a fat strain of animals through breeding
practices. Farmers and cattlemen have breeding down to a science.
They can, with considerable precision, obtain the body composition
they desire in their bulls, cows, hogs, and chickens. Since we can't
control breeding practices in humans, the situation is much harder
to study and we must use more roundabout strategies to show the
influence of heredity.

When we examine the correlation of body weights between parents and their children, we can observe that obesity does seem to
run in families. If both parents are obese, the probability that any
given child will also be obese is about 8 in 10. If only one parent
is obese it drops to 4 in 10, while if both parents are lean it drops
to 1 in 10.

However, a comparison of children with their parents does not
separate the influence of heredity from that of the environment. It
could all be due to eating patterns in these families.

Other more sophisticated strategies for studying this phenomenon are not open to the same criticism. When identical twins are
compared with fraternal twins of the same sex, the correlation between the body weights of identical twins and their amounts of body
fat is much higher, even if the twins have been raised in different
environments. Identical twins, who share the same heredity, have
body weights that vary, on the average, by around 3 pounds. That
3-pound variation is due to environmental influences. Fraternal
twins do not share the same heredity, and the difference between
their body weights jumps up to around 8 or 9 pounds. In other
words, when environmental influences alone are operating, you get
a 3-pound difference, but when you add a difference in heredity to
the environmental influence, the difference increases almost three-
fold—up to 8 or 9 pounds. This has led many researchers to estimate that between 50 and 80 percent of the variability in body
weight in our population is due to hereditary factors.[4-7]

Of course, any variability in the body weight of a single individual, in your weight or in mine, will be due to environmental causes.
Hereditary influences are determined by the time we are born, and,
as I have said before, all you have to do is compare your body build
with that of your ancestors to determine whether you have a genetic

predisposition to accumulate fat more easily than a naturally slim person.

Because it has been customary to downplay, if not completely ignore, the role of heredity in our weight problems, and because this has led to the false belief that it should be simple to control your body weight by dieting, many overweight people have carried around an awful lot of unnecessary guilt. And, because so many "experts" do not appreciate the genetic contribution and how it responds to dieting, the situation becomes even more monstrous when you realize that the diet "cures" they prescribe only end up increasing the original predisposition to store fat!

The genetic influence on body weight is approached from another vantage point by recent research on set-point theory.

Set-Point Theory

In 1982, William Bennett and Joel Gurin published a remarkable book (*The Dieter's Dilemma*) in which they explored the concept of a "set point" in determining body weight.[8] After reviewing scores of studies involving both humans and animals, they concluded that individuals have a biological set point that determines body weight "when we are not thinking about it." That is, genetic predispositions lead to a particular body chemistry that determines the amount of lean and fat tissue in our bodies. When we try to change our body weights, adaptive responses occur that work against the change and try to preserve the status quo. Even if we succeed, the moment we deviate from the dietary or exercise regimen aimed at changing our weight we return quickly and easily to the weight and body composition to which our set points have been programmed.

On first examination, the evidence appears quite convincing. When normally skinny people agree to overeat for research purposes, they find it rather hard to gain weight. They gain only a fraction of the weight they should theoretically gain if all the extra calories they eat were stored as fat. Somehow, the body elevates its metabolic rate and burns off most of the excess calories that the subjects force themselves to eat. And (I know this may be hard to believe) skinny people often become as uncomfortable trying to overeat to gain weight as fat people do undereating to lose! When these experimental overeaters return to their preferred intakes, body weights return to normal quite quickly.

And, as we know all too well, the same thing occurs in reverse for undereating. People do not lose the same number of calories out of their fat cells as would be predicted from a cutback in their diets. Metabolism slows. When normal eating is resumed, weight is quickly regained because, in addition to your lowered metabolic needs, the fat-storing hormones and enzymes become more active. It doesn't matter whether you are fat or thin to begin with: after using a low-calorie diet, weight is quickly regained when you return to your normal intake.

According to Bennett and Gurin, persons with "high" set points are naturally fat, while persons with "low" set points are naturally thin. And they will remain that way unless continuous, strenuous efforts are made to alter the situation.

It is hard to imagine a more gloomy outlook for the person who would like to lose some weight, keep it off, and establish a low set point when his or her constitution says high! Fortunately, that feeling results from a misperception of the realities in the situation.

Bennett and Gurin suggest that the only way to change your set point may be through physical activity. I am in general agreement with that view, but also believe that the nature of the American diet, high in fat and processed foods, makes it easier for the body to store fat than a diet *low* in fat and *high* in complex carbohydrates. Animal studies show that diets high in fat and sugar can lead to an increased number of fat cells (hyperplasia).[9] In addition, as I explained in the first part of this book, calories being equal, your body will not convert as many of them to fat when more of those calories come from high-fiber foods with little fat content.[10]

Part of the pessimism generated from set-point theory is due to a misinterpretation of the real meaning of "set point." The word itself suggests a "point" that is primarily determined by your heredity.

The truth of the matter is that your genetic predispositions establish a *range* of weight that is affected by what and how you eat, and by your level of physical activity. Whatever you weigh results from an adaptive interaction between your heredity and your eating and activity behaviors. I am going to show you the evidence from both animal and human studies that proves that permanent changes, *both up and down,* can be made in your set point as a result of what you eat and how active you are. Once the hormone and enzyme changes have become established at your new weight, your body will work to protect that new weight from changing just as it did the old.

What Makes the Difference in Our Basic Tendencies?

Differences in our dispositions toward obesity and in our adaptive responses to diet and exercise may be due to a variety of physiological and biochemical mechanisms. Any one of them, or various combinations, may be operative in any individual case. Thus, while it is quite correct to say that obesity can only develop when there is an excess of energy intake over expenditure, *the excess of available energy need not occur because a person is EATING MORE than the average person.*

Some bodies are much more efficient than others and simply do not need as much fuel.

Some bodies, but not all, may have a way of *preventing* fat accumulation by turning on a fat burner as soon as an excess of calories enters the system. One study with rats showed that this may happen in some cases after a single big meal.[11] It may happen in other organisms only after the animal (or person) has overeaten a considerable amount for several days.

I will explain how several of the most important mechanisms work.

Thermogenesis and the Thermic Effect

Approximately 40 percent of the energy in our food is actually captured and transformed into the form of energy we need to maintain bodily processes. The rest is never absorbed or given off as heat in the process called thermogenesis. Body cells of average-weight people appear to give off more heat than the body cells of fat people. This means that more of the food energy is being "wasted" in thinner people; their cells are inefficient.

In one study, the difference in the average amount of heat given off by the cells of twelve normal-weight persons in comparison with the average of fourteen overweight persons was very large, as you can see in Figure 19-1. In fact, *only one* of fourteen obese persons in the study had fat tissue that produced as much heat as any of the twelve average-weight persons who had participated. The energy that's being conserved by the overweight persons is available for storage, and may be contributing to their obesity.[12]

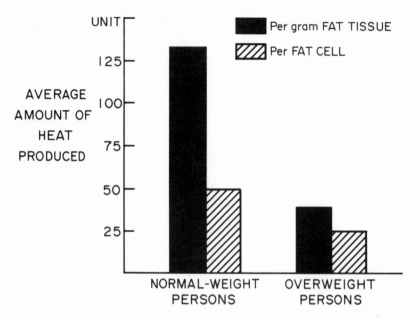

FIGURE 19-1.   Average amount of heat produced per gram of fat tissue and per fat cell in normal-weight and overweight persons. Overweight persons have much larger fat cells, so, while in the cellular comparison the average-weight persons are producing twice as much heat, when the comparison is between equal amounts of tissue —per gram—they are seen to produce three times as much. (The numbers along the vertical axis refer to minute units of heat energy.)

Each time a person eats, a certain amount of energy is required for the metabolic processes that convert the nutrients in food into the form needed by our bodies. The extra heat that's produced during digestion is called the "thermic effect of food." While the evidence is still controversial, some studies show that average-weight people may have a thermic effect of food that is almost twice as great as overweight persons, and that some overweight persons may have little or no thermic effect at all. The thermic effect in thin persons may increase their metabolic rate by over 10 percent.[13]

When persons go on a low-calorie diet, the thermic effect of food may be drastically diminished. It disappears, of course, on a starvation diet. This leads to an automatic reduction in metabolic needs of about 10 percent since your body no longer has to work at metabolizing your food.

The Sodium Pump

A major portion of the energy used by your body, perhaps between 20 and 40 percent of your total basal metabolic needs, is involved with one very important process—keeping the correct balance between sodium and potassium on the insides and outsides of trillions of body cells. Speaking somewhat figuratively, there appear to be tiny pumps on our cell membranes, and each time one particular enzyme operates (sodium, potassium-ATPase) a certain amount of sodium is shoved out of the cell, and a certain amount of potassium enters. It is important to keep the concentration of sodium within the cells lower than in the surrounding fluid—hence the name "sodium pump."

Obese rodents have less enzyme activity and evidently fewer active pumps on their cell membranes, which would lead to less energy being used in sodium pump activity. This is also reflected in lower thermogenesis in these animals.[14-16]

Human studies are just beginning to appear, and while the results are still controversial, two studies have shown a decrease in sodium pump activity in red blood cells from overweight individuals, which can decrease metabolic needs by several hundred calories a day if other tissue acted similarly. However, another study using liver tissue showed just the reverse, so the question of generality is not settled.[17,18]

Sodium pump activity may be a major source of the thermic effect discussed above, and the more active these pumps are, the greater the amount of thermogenesis. Since sodium pump activity uses so much of the body's resting energy needs, rather small differences in the efficiency of this mechanism could contribute to obesity.

Brown Adipose Tissue

Many mammals, including human beings, have a small amount of "brown" fat that functions quite differently from ordinary "white" fat. Brown fat is highly active—it burns calories like a furnace under certain conditions. While a pound of white fat may need only 4 or 5 calories a day to stay alive, a pound of brown fat has the capacity to burn several hundred calories an hour!

In normal, nonobese rodents, brown fat turns on when the animal is subjected to a cold environment or when it is overfed. While brown fat accounts for only 1 to 2 percent of body weight in these animals, when it becomes highly active it may account for 60 percent of the body's heat production. It grows tremendously in mass in response to cold in order to turn out more heat, and in response to overfeeding in order to burn off the extra calories. That is, in rodents that are not normally fat, and rather hard to fatten, brown fat increases in mass and in activity (including increased sodium pump activity) when these animals are given highly tempting diets of peanut butter, chocolate bars, salami, sweetened milk, etc. By increasing thermogenesis, the brown fat can waste two-thirds of the ingested calories.[19-21] At least one study has shown an increase in the activity of already existing brown fat cells after a single big meal.[11]

When the tempting diets are removed, the brown fat stays active in the normal, nonobese animal until regular weight is achieved.

Genetically obese rodents have a defect in brown fat.

It doesn't turn on in response to cold. In spite of having more ordinary fat as insulation on their bodies, they will die at temperatures to which normal rodents can adapt.

And, in the obese rodents, brown fat doesn't increase in mass or turn on and start to burn calories in response to overfeeding.[22]

The existence of functional brown fat in the human body has been verified in locations similar to those found in animals, such as between the shoulder blades and around our internal organs. It seems to be responsive to the same central nervous system chemicals that stimulate it in rodents. For example, the temperature of the skin on our backs in the region of the brown fat goes up under the influence of ephedrine.

The direct investigation of brown fat generally requires operative techniques that are not possible with humans, so further investigation of its role in predispositions to obesity, and how it adapts to help the naturally lean preserve body weight on high-calorie diets, will have to await the development of a suitable methodology.

Adipode Tissue Lipoprotein Lipase

Adipose tissue lipoprotein lipase (AT-LPL) is an enzyme that resides on the walls of our fat cells. It controls the rate at which triglycerides circulating in the bloodstream are broken down into fatty acids and transported into the cells for storage.

AT-LPL is significantly more active on the fat cells of overweight people and genetically obese rodents. In those Zucker rats that I mentioned previously, heightened AT-LPL activity occurs just prior to the onset of obesity and seems to cause it.[23]

This enzyme may prove to have an important role in human obesity. It may contribute to its initial cause, and it may contribute to the rapid weight gain that occurs after a low-calorie diet.

When research subjects were put on a low-calorie diet, the activity of this enzyme decreased since there was less need to transport fat into the fat cells each day. However, the enzyme activity during the diet decreased *less* over time for overweight subjects than for normal-weight subjects.[24,25] In other words, the fat cells of the overweight subjects were still actively transporting more fat across their membranes than were the cells of the normal-weight persons, during the diet. This may help explain the resistance to weight loss seen in some overweight persons.

However, the most important role that AT-LPL may play in preserving obesity may lie in its reaction to a resumption of normal food intake following a low-calorie diet. After a 600-calorie formula diet on which male volunteers had lost approximately 35 pounds, AT-LPL activity was elevated to more than four times its pre-diet level. Four of the subjects were followed for 8 to 14 months after the diet. Three of the subjects had regained weight to the point where they were *105* percent of their pre-diet weight. In these subjects, AT-LPL had returned to near-normal levels, though it was still slightly higher than pre-diet levels. However, in the one subject who had kept off most of the weight lost during the experiment by continuing to restrain his food intake, AT-LPL activity remained markedly elevated. It was as though his fat cells were continuing their effort to "pull" the calories out of his bloodstream.[26]

Other Mechanisms That Influence Obesity

When you go to your physician for a checkup and he does your "blood-work," he may check your thyroid function. The thyroid hormone plays a major role in energy utilization, and, if your levels are low, it is obvious that your metabolic needs are reduced. Perhaps 5 percent of the obese population have significantly reduced thyroid function. If you deviate by only 10 or 20 percent from average, your thyroid function may still be considered normal. However, even this deviation may mean that you need several hundred calories less each day to maintain body weight than does the average person.

If your thyroid function appears normal, your physician may assume that you are eating too much and need to go on a diet.

If your physician has not been keeping up with recent advances in obesity research and puts you on a diet of fewer than 1200 calories, you should be sure to show him this and the following chapters. He should already know that such diets will *decrease* thyroid activity still further. When you go on a low-calorie diet, in particular one of the low-carbohydrate types, the conversion of thyroid into its active form, triiodothyronine (T_3), is reduced, your ability to burn calories is reduced, and this is reflected in a lowering of metabolic rate.[27]

But, in addition to thyroid activity, there are many, many other biochemical factors that can affect your body weight and your ability to store or utilize energy. So far I have discussed just four of the most important mechanisms. I will briefly note a few of the others so that you can appreciate the complexity of the situation.

Insulin affects your ability to incorporate energy into your cells. A high insulin level means increased fat-storage tendencies and may be a precursor to adult onset diabetes. When you go on a diet, your body cells become more sensitive to insulin and blood insulin levels fall. That's marvelous when you consider the beneficial effects that result when you reduce blood sugar and insulin levels, but it also means that when you finish your diet, the transport of energy into your more sensitive fat cells will be greatly facilitated—up perhaps two or three times its previous rate.[28]

The catecholamines and growth hormone affect your ability to burn fat. Low levels, or a decreased sensitivity on the part of your body cells to the fat-mobilizing effect of these hormones, mean a decreased ability to burn calories. The catecholamines also have a direct, elevating effect on metabolic rate, which seems to be somewhat less in overweight people.[29]

Many enzymes are involved as catalysts in breaking down the fat and carbohydrate in your diet for use as immediate energy or for storage. Many others are involved in taking it from storage and transforming it for use as energy. You can be on the high side for fat storage, or on the low side for energy breakdown. Or, if you are really unfortunate, in the wrong direction on both.[30]

The body has various routes through which it can either waste or conserve energy. In what is called the "glycerol phosphate shuttle," one route produces 50 percent more usable energy than another, more wasteful route. When people go on diets, they begin to use the route that produces the most usable energy (the less wasteful route) in order to conserve calories. The shuttle is of great interest, and is worth further investigation, because, even along the wasteful route, there is a gate, or trap: in one direction the energy can be shunted off for conversion to fat, whereas in the other direction it is converted to the high-energy form for immediate use. Research suggests that fat people may be more predisposed to use the conservation or fat-storage route.[31,32]

In the breakdown of stored sugar (glycolysis) there is also a pathway in which the body can waste energy. It is called a "futile cycle." When stored energy enters the futile cycle, body cells shuffle the fuel back and forth from its storage to a more usable form, wasting a portion as they do this, but not producing any work. The cells seem to be acting like a car with a high idle speed, burning much of its stored fuel, but not going anywhere.[33,34]

The body's cells may also cycle, or break down and rebuild their protein components, at variable rates. These rates may be influenced by hereditary factors, diet, and exercise. Higher rates of turnover will require more energy.[35]

All of the mechanisms that I have discussed can predispose a person toward obesity if they are at levels that facilitate fat storage or interfere with the conversion of stored fuel into its usable forms. You cannot, unfortunately, determine your own predispositions because most of these mechanisms can only be studied in advanced research laboratories.

But the measurement of all of these mechanisms is not important to the matter at hand. I have described them in some detail so that you will have a better idea of the many biochemical processes that are operating in your own body, and the patience to go about cultivating changes that make weight control easier, rather than more difficult.

What *is* important is that we know low-calorie dieting will turn on an adaptive reaction in one or more of the mechanisms I have described in an attempt to *save* calories and preserve body weight. This only makes weight control more difficult.

We also know that physical activity will *turn on* one or more of these mechanisms to *facilitate energy utilization and reduce the amount that must be stored in your fat cells.* This makes weight control easier.

This remarkable ability of our bodies to respond to life-style factors—changes in diet and exercise—is what "metabolic adaptation" is all about.

In the next chapter I describe a few of the most dramatic illustrations of metabolic adaptation.

20

METABOLIC EFFECTS OF DIETARY CHANGES

When naturally slim people agree to eat several thousand calories more each day than they would normally eat, for research purposes, one or more of the mechanisms I have just described—such as sodium pump or thyroid activity, futile cycling, the glycerol phosphate shuttle, perhaps brown fat activity—speeds up. Then, just sitting still, these volunteers can begin to burn from 15 to 50 percent more calories, around the clock.[1]

When overweight people go on a fast or low-calorie diet, one or more of the energy control mechanisms slows down, and these persons may burn between 30 and 45 percent fewer calories each day—around the clock.[2,3]

Almost all persons will have a dramatic metabolic slowdown when they cut their calories in half, and it seems to be an almost invariable occurrence on diets of 800 or fewer calories.[4,5] But some persons may make adjustments to very small deviations.

For example, in a classic study reported over 80 years ago, Neumann[6] compared his weight changes during carefully controlled variations up to several hundred calories above and below his normal intake. After gaining or losing just a few pounds, his weight would level off and remain stable for a prolonged period of time when theoretically he should have gained or lost 20 or 30 pounds. He evidently did not vary his physical activity. When he increased intake, some mechanism seemed to speed up his metabolism and burned his excess calories. When he cut back, his metabolism apparently slowed to conserve energy.

In Neumann's carefully controlled case, the statement appearing in almost all diet books that increasing or decreasing caloric intake by 100 calories a day means a yearly weight gain or loss of 10 pounds did not hold true.

I believe there are many people similar to Professor Neumann. When physical activity is held constant, deviations in caloric intake of from 100 to several hundred calories lead to some small losses or gains. Then weight levels off as the body's chemistry adapts. This phenomenon has led some researchers to propose that energy needs are controlled by an "autoregulatory homeostatic" mechanism: if you eat more, your body will use nutrients less efficiently; if you eat less, it will use them more efficiently.[7] Thus, you can vary your caloric intake up or down by several hundred calories each day, and, over a period of weeks, be several hundred higher or lower than your measurable energy expenditure. But, because of this self-regulating mechanism, which determines how efficiently you will use calories, you will not gain or lose any weight (except for fluctuations in your water balance).

This autoregulatory theory appears to be an arithmetic or statistical way of expressing the idea of "set point" that I discussed in the preceding chapter. Simply put, it seems that your body has a way of counting calories without your awareness. Normally you may use about 40 percent of your intake to support metabolic processes, and waste the rest in heat or the process of elimination. If you increase your intake, the body becomes less efficient, using perhaps 30 or 35 percent of your intake. If you cut calories, it may increase your efficiency to 45 or 50 percent. Of course, a change in one or another of the biochemical mechanisms I have previously discussed (or one not yet discovered) must underlie this more statistical description of the regulatory process.

Another classic study, this one done over 60 years ago, clearly shows how this regulatory system comes into play after a period of dieting. And, what is perhaps more important, the results of the study suggest that one may gain a resistance to weight loss and a need to eat fewer and fewer calories to maintain a given weight the more one "practices" dieting. Benedict et al.[8] recruited a group of volunteers who agreed to cut calories by about one-third for a prolonged period of time. Within 9 weeks, following a loss of about 18 pounds, the body weights of the participants reached a plateau. Metabolic rate had slowed by about 20 percent. The subjects were given times out from their diets at Thanksgiving and Christmas and could eat as they pleased. Even at Christmas, with 2 weeks off, metabolic rate recovered only about half way to baseline. Each time the subjects went back on their diets, after Thanksgiving and Christmas, *their metabolic rates dropped more quickly than the first time.* In spite of continued adherence, no weight was lost during the last several weeks of dieting. When the subjects returned to eating freely again, they regained weight about three times faster than they had lost it.

I quote these classic studies because much of the basic knowledge of metabolic adaptation has been available to health professionals for a considerable period of time. However, we have not paid much attention to the implications of this early research for weight control.

Present-day research with animals clearly shows the very striking and rapid adaptation that can occur to extreme deprivation, such as a total fast. DiGirolamo et al.[9] fasted a group of rats for 3 days, in which time they lost about 10 percent of their body weight. He found that it took only 60 percent of their pre-diet intake to maintain their weight for 13 days afterward. To continue weight loss required a reduction to 40 percent of their prior caloric needs.

Rats have higher energy needs per pound of body weight than humans and tend to have a life expectancy of about 3 to 4 years. By comparison, one might expect the aftereffects of fasting to last much longer in people when they have lost 10 percent of their body weight via the starvation route. It takes about 10 days to 2 weeks for a human to lose 10 percent of body weight on a fast, and the reduced caloric needs are likely to last a proportionately longer time. Judging from the eating records that have been kept for me by persons who have used low-calorie diets, I would estimate that caloric requirements for weight maintenance may be reduced to about 60 or 70 percent of normal for as much as several months.[10]

Many lifelong dieters claim that it gets harder and harder to lose weight with each succeeding diet, especially after they have lost weight on a fast, put it all back on again, and then try the more healthy route of moderate caloric restriction.

In order to investigate the possibility that extreme forms of dieting might make it more difficult to lose weight on anything but diets extremely low in calories, Dr. H. C. Meng, professor of physiology at the Vanderbilt Medical School, and I devised an animal study to determine whether repeated fasting on the part of obese rats would give them practice in resisting weight loss on the animal equivalent of a sensible diet. This would give us some evidence that the feast or famine, binge/fast approach that some people use to control their weight might only make it more difficult to lose on a "sensible" weight management diet.

We matched two groups of rats on initial body weights. Then we allowed one group to eat freely on what is called a "supermarket" diet.[11] Each day we gave them a variety of foods from a list that included peanut butter, chocolate bars and chocolate chip cookies, salami, cheese, marshmallows, sweetened milk, etc. On the average, over a 108-day period, this group of rats increased body weight by 30 percent, in spite of the fact that we were using a strain of rats that is not predisposed to obesity (Sprague-Dawleys).

The other group was given the same tempting assortment of foods, but every 15, 20, or 25 days they fasted for 3 days. Although they fasted four times in this period, they ate enough on the other days to end up weighing approximately as much as the non-fasted group.

Then came our test. Would the animals that had "practice" conserving calories through fasting and then quickly regaining weight on a fattening diet lose weight at the same rate as the equally fat, but never-fasted group, when we put both of them on standard low-fat laboratory fare once again (our rat version of a "sensible" weight-loss diet)?

The results were dramatic.

The weight-loss curves for the two groups of rats when they were put on our rat version of a sensible weight-loss diet appear to support human experience. The group that had never "tried to control" its weight by fasting lost 51 percent more weight within 15 days compared with the group that had been given practice in fasting. Apparently, very much in line with the anecdotal reports of people who have spent a lifetime dieting, weight loss proceeds much more slowly in rats that have been subjected to repeated fasting in comparison with rats that have never fasted before.

The weight-loss curves for the two different groups are presented in Figure 20-1.[12]

But some fattened rats (unfortunately like some overweight people) may never lose any weight at all on a "sensible" diet! Rolls,

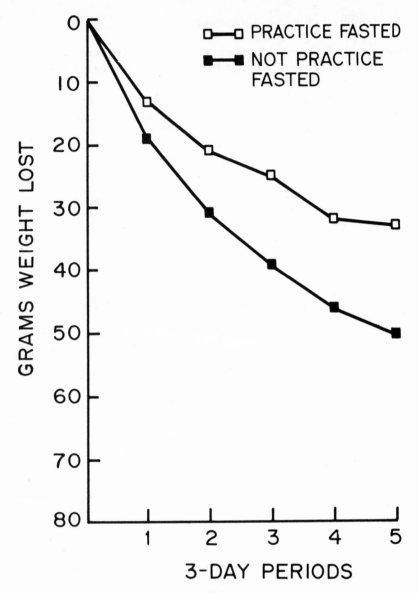

FIGURE 20-1. Comparison of weight-loss curves for "supermarket"-fed rats that had either been practice fasted or not practiced fasted after gaining weight on a supermarket diet. Rats that had never fasted lost 51 percent more weight than the practiced fasted when they returned to eating standard laboratory chow. (From Katahn and Meng.[12])

Rowe, and Turner fed hooded rats on the "supermarket" diet for a prolonged period and found that normal weight would not be reinstated no matter how long the animals were subsequently kept on regular chow.[13] Evidently, overeating on high fat and sweetened foods had brought about some physiological change that was not reversible on a return to a normal diet. The mechanisms underlying this rather startling phenomenon are not yet understood, but are under investigation in our own and other laboratories.

The research I have discussed in this chapter leads to several conclusions and speculations:

1. Normally nonobese animals, just like humans, will overeat and fatten if tasty high-fat and high-sugar foods are freely available.

2. In the process of gaining weight on such diets, some animals, and possibly some humans, may experience alterations in fundamental biochemical processes that make weight loss and weight maintenance on a sensible diet more difficult.

3. Low-calorie dieting elicits a metabolic response that serves to protect the body against weight loss.

4. A repetitive pattern of feasting on a high-fat, high-sugar diet, followed by fasting, may increase an organism's ability to maintain obesity on fewer and fewer calories.[14]

Let's now take a look at the effects of physical activity.

21

METABOLIC EFFECTS OF PHYSICAL ACTIVITY

Writing in the *International Journal of Obesity,* P. J. Bradley[1] succinctly summarized the effects of physical activity on weight management in a single sentence:

". . . exercise does more than utilize energy. It can depress appetite, relieve psychological stress, prevent insulin resistance, depress the resting serum insulin level, facilitate peripheral T_3 metabolism, augment thermogenesis, increase lean body mass, and increase the carbohydrate handling capacity [p. 46]."

Indeed, the number of health-related benefits of physical activity can be extended beyond this already lengthy list to include a reduction in mild hypertension, lowering of serum triglycerides, resistance to bone deterioration that accompanies aging, and an increase in the HDL to LDL (high- to low-density lipoprotein) cholesterol ratio that may offer some protection against cardiovascular disease.

However, my main concern is with the weight-related benefits of physical activity, especially when done in accordance with Metabolic Breakthrough principles. I have made some claims about the superior weight-control value of those activities that require moving your whole body in continuous rather than sporadic movements. I have also insisted that such activities must be done almost every day, and that even modest increases in muscle mass will increase your fat-burning power.

My analysis of fifty-five different studies of the effects of physical training illustrates that, when you follow the principles of the Metabolic Breakthrough Activity Program, your body will

1. automatically adapt to the new demands you are placing on it by losing weight,

2. burn off an even larger amount of fat than your scale may show, and

3. increase its round-the-clock fat-burning power by a slight addition to its active muscle mass.

In early 1983, Dr. Jack Wilmore[2] published a report in which he listed, study by study, the body weight and body composition changes (amounts of lean and fat tissue changes) that occurred as a result of physical training in fifty-five different research projects. The studies included men and women of all ages up to the late fifties and covered activities such as walking and jogging, bicycling, calisthenics, strength training, and a variety of competitive sports. Only five of the studies employed persons who were significantly overweight, and it was physical activity, not dieting, that was being investigated.

Dr. Wilmore's tabulation of the results of so many individual studies gave me the opportunity to examine the changes in weight, muscle mass, and fat mass that would occur naturally in response to physical training, whether or not weight loss was the desired objective.

These are the questions I wanted to answer:

1. Did some of the activities lead to more weight loss and fat loss?

2. Did males and females change in the same way and degree?

3. Did number of times per week make a significant difference?

4. Were changes in the amount of muscle gained related to the amount of fat lost?

5. Did it seem that participants increased their food intake to compensate for the energy needed by their higher level of activity?

I entered the data from all of the individual studies into the computer and performed a variety of statistical analyses.

These are the answers I obtained:

1. Walking, jogging, and bicycling resulted in significantly more weight loss and fat loss than all other activities.

2. Females lost just as much weight and body fat as a function of physical activity, but ONLY IN WALKING, JOGGING, AND BICYCLING, not in other activities.

3. Number of times per week was important. Four or more was

related to significantly more weight loss and fat loss than three or fewer.

4. The more muscle gained, the greater the fat loss.

5. Previously sedentary people do not appear to increase food intake to compensate for all of the energy expended in physical activity.

These results deserve a little discussion and amplification.

Continuous walking, jogging, and bicycling are the most efficient ways for the average person to burn calories. Even among athletes, working out at competitive intensities, no intermittent activity is likely to equal or exceed the caloric needs of continuous activity. For example, hour for hour, tennis will not equal the requirements of cross-country running. Thus, I anticipated that all continuous whole-body activities would cause the greatest weight and fat losses. (There were not enough studies to separate out swimming for comparison, but I have already pointed out on page 53 that, while swimming is an excellent whole-body activity, weight and fat losses tend not to be as great as with other whole-body activities.)

Because of initial differences in lean tissue mass and hormone secretions, I expected males to lose more weight than females, and to build more muscle mass as a result of physical activity. It's no secret that women will lose weight more slowly on diets, and I expected that similar tendencies might be present as a result of physical activity. I am glad to say that this did not prove to be true. While women lost a bit less weight and less fat, and gained a bit less lean tissue in activities such as calisthenics, strength training, and field sports, *there was no difference when it came to walking, jogging, and bicycling.*

The more muscle gained, the greater the fat loss. Now, this is an important point. Muscle is active tissue. If you build muscle tissue, you burn more calories round the clock. My analysis showed that people who were exercising at an intensity that would build muscle —actually *adding* some muscle weight to their bodies—ended up *losing more of their body fat* than people who were not exercising in a way that added to their muscle tissue. There is a direct relationship between the intensity of activity and the degree of muscle tissue you build. This is another illustration of the importance of the Metabolic Breakthrough Intensity principle during continuous whole-body movement for purposes of weight control. When you move briskly at that 70 to 90 percent of maximum heart rate, which is precisely the training intensity used in the studies I examined, you build more muscle tissue than you do in leisurely movement.

And now for what is perhaps the most important finding when it comes to using physical activity as an aid during weight loss as well as maintenance:

Do people tend to eat more as they get active, when they are not thinking about it and have not engaged in an activity program for purposes of weight control?

Exercisers did not compensate for the increased energy needs of activity even though subjects in fifty of the studies did not participate for weight-control reasons.

In the natural course of adaptation to activity:

exercisers lost approximately one pound of fat for every ten hours of exercise,
and gained about a quarter of a pound of muscle tissue for every ten hours of exercise.

This means that, in becoming more active, exercisers used about 350 calories an hour out of their fat cells, which was not replaced through increased food intake. If it were, there would have been no change in either weight or fat loss.

On the average, the studies lasted about 16 weeks and involved less than 40 hours of activity. Certainly, over a long period, the body would reach a new level of adaptation, balancing caloric intake with energy expenditure. Just as in the Stanford study, discussed on page 61, it is likely that any exerciser will end up eating more and weighing less in the long run.

In the present series of studies it is only possible to make a guess about caloric intake. Since these were physical training studies aimed at increasing cardiovascular endurance or other aspects of conditioning related to sports and activity, it is likely that the minimum intensity was at least 70 percent of maximum heart rate during the major portion of activity. Activities such as brisk walking or jogging at this intensity will use between 400 and 600 calories an hour. However, as I indicated above, the average fat loss was equal to about 350 calories per hour. Thus, even during the period of weight loss, participants in these physical training studies probably *increased* their caloric intake by at least 50, and probably something more like 150 or 250, calories a day *and still lost weight.*

If they had not increased intake over their pre-program levels, they would have lost even more weight. But my point is that, with the freedom to eat as they pleased in almost all studies, *the appetite did not increase to keep pace with the extra physical activity.* Instead, it seemed to adapt at a level of intake about 350 calories below daily needs for at least an average of 16 weeks.

Will this hold true for people who are significantly overweight?

There is strong evidence that it will for at least several weeks, or until surplus fat stores are lost. It occurs even when *no* effort is made to go on a diet and reduce body weight.

Woo et al.[3] surreptitiously measured the calorie intake of six obese women who averaged 202.6 pounds, or 167 percent of ideal weight. These women had voluntarily entered a metabolic ward for study during weight maintenance, not weight loss. In three different 19-day periods they were asked to remain sedentary or walk on a treadmill for either a short or a long period of time each day.

When they walked for about 40 minutes a day, increasing their total metabolic needs by about 10 percent, *they ate about 114 fewer calories per day than their maintenance requirements.*

When they exercised for about 90 minutes a day, increasing their daily needs by about 25 percent, *they ate 369 fewer calories per day than their actual daily expenditure.*

The same investigators also studied the long-term relationship of food intake, exercise, and weight change for 57 days in another group of three women whose weight averaged 221 pounds.[4] Once again they found that with an increase of daily energy needs by 25 percent as a result of extra walking the women did not compensate by eating more. The researchers made no attempt to put these women on a diet, but instead provided unlimited palatable food, "simply" prepared. On the average, the women lost about 2 pounds per week without dieting.

The conclusions you should draw from this analysis are that almost-daily walking or jogging at Metabolic Breakthrough Intensity is your best bet to facilitate fat loss and build fat-burning muscle mass and that, while you are doing so, there will be a natural tendency *not* to compensate with an increase in appetite.

And perhaps the best news I can give you is that women appear to do about as well as men when they follow Metabolic Breakthrough principles instead of dieting.

22

THE TRANSITION TO MAINTENANCE: CASE HISTORIES AND RECOMMENDATIONS

Before I answer the question, "What Does It Take?" I want to answer another: "What will it take if you *don't* follow the principles of the Metabolic Breakthrough Plan?"

In the fall of 1982 I went to three of the most successful commercial weight-loss programs and asked them to collaborate with me in a research project.[1]

I said, "Show me your *successful* cases. I want to see what people who have reached their desired weights using your program are doing to keep it off."

All of these programs advertised rather extensively, and made it a point that they were "weight loss without uncomfortable, strenuous exercise" programs.

I want to make it clear that this was not a project to evaluate specific commercial programs. My purpose was to look at the follow-up results with respect to specific *caloric intakes* during dieting, when physical activity, which might counter the effects of metabolic adaptation, was not required.

Two of the programs I investigated used diets of approximately 800 calories, while one used a formula with fewer than 350 calories per day.

Unfortunately, none of these programs had long-term follow-up data. However, they were able to show me their maintenance plans and some individual records of people during the first year after the diet. Successful women were eating approximately 1200 to 1300 calories a day, and men between 1600 and 1800. In the case of the formula plan, I was able to obtain individual weekly eating and activity records, including pedometer readings for physical activity, to verify these figures.

Not one of these persons had adopted a consistently active life-style, although a few were participating in an occasional dance class or a weekend sport.

These "maintenance intakes" are about 30 to 40 percent below average. *Most people will lose at least a pound a week on such maintenance plans.* But not an inactive person who has become metabolically adapted to a low-calorie intake.

In case you number yourself among such persons, let me say immediately that you are not stuck for life with such low maintenance requirements.

In this chapter I want to show you what a few persons who have kept large amounts of weight off for over five years are doing to keep it off. I also will give you some data from our large-scale follow-ups.

Then, in Chapters 26 and 27 I will show you what *you* can do to recover from the effects of low-calorie dieting and increase your food intake to normal levels without regaining the weight you have worked so hard to lose.

Figure 22-1 presents the complete range of variation in the adult lives of five persons whose biological predispositions, given their previously sedentary lives, established what Bennett and Gurin refer to as a "set point" at the top of the depicted range when eating without restraint. Present weights are indicated by the crossbars at the lower ends of the ranges.

The first woman (over 40 pounds lighter than her highest weight six years ago) averages approximately 1860 calories per day, adding about 4 miles of either walking or jogging to the baseline require-ments of about 2 miles of movement in her work and other respon-sibilities.

The second woman (over 50 pounds lighter) maintains her weight at about 1915 calories, provided she adds 20 minutes every day of continuous freestyle swimming to an otherwise sedentary existence. Hers is one instance in which swimming has proved to be an excellent calorie-burning activity. But her records also illustrate another very important point: *the moment she stops swimming, she gains*

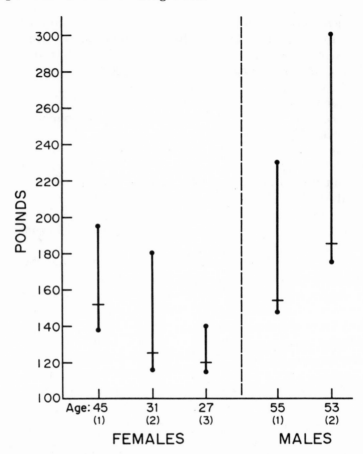

FIGURE 22-1.   Present weights (crossbars) and complete range of weights during their adult lives of five individuals who have kept large amounts of weight off for at least five years with physical activity levels that meet Metabolic Breakthrough standards. See the text for an explanation.

weight almost as fast as an inactive person who deviates from a low-calorie dieter's maintenance plan.

The third woman maintains herself at about 1905 calories, averaging about 7 miles of walking every day. She fits this activity in by walking 1½ miles to work, and taking a half-hour walk at lunch. Her eating records are very interesting to me because she likes candy and has at least one bar every day, plus one other dessert food. But she always has those eight servings of grains, vegetables, and fruit as well, to be sure that she has an otherwise nutritious diet.

These data are obtained from eating and activity diaries kept as part of our follow-up research from a select group of former participants each year since the Vanderbilt program began in 1976.

Today, these three women all fall within normal limits of energy needs, *provided* they add the amount of activity that might have been required of them in their daily lives a few generations ago. Without that level of activity there is no doubt that their caloric needs at desirable weight would be reduced to the levels (1200 to 1300) required for persons who have used low-calorie diets and who are presently relying on dietary restriction for weight control.

The eating diaries of these women show no particular restraint in eating except after "big weekends." All three are at the present time attractive single women, and they are, frankly, not spending their weekend evenings at home. While they are all eating a basically nutritious diet, there are still plenty of cocktails, peanuts, candy, and occasional rich desserts in these records. Fluctuations of 2 or 3 pounds are normal, but none of them seems to be required to cut back to fewer than 1200 calories for more than one or two days to get back to her desired weight.

The first male illustrated in the figure once weighed 230 pounds. I know this person rather well. It's myself. As I mentioned earlier, my "set-point" range seemed to have an upper boundry at around 230 pounds 20 years go when I ate freely without any physical activity. Today, at 154 pounds, my eating and activity records show 2960 calories per day (more than I ate when I was sedentary) with 35 to 40 miles of jogging each week and tennis once or twice a week. My job as a college professor is sedentary, and without extra physical activity my pedometer shows that I rarely exceed 2 miles per day of walking. However, my extra recreational activity puts my daily caloric requirements several hundred calories higher than that of the average inactive male between 35 and 55 years of age.

The second male provides an example of what it might take in the way of physical activity for persons with extreme tendencies toward obesity. This man is one of a *small* number of folks whom I call my "weight-loss heroes." There are not many massively obese persons who have lost 125 pounds or more and *never* regained at least a good part of their earlier weight.

This second male has a very high "set-point range." He lost 125

pounds on an 1800-calorie diet combined with what most overweight persons would consider an unbelievable increase in physical
activity. He maintains his present weight on approximately 2600
calories per day and a weekly average of (hold your breath):

35 miles of jogging,
4 hours of racquet ball,
5 hours of an exercise bicycle, and
1½ hours of weight training.

I'm not done. He no longer drives to work or to appointments
near his office and averages about 5 miles per day of additional
walking. He has the sort of genetic predisposition toward obesity
that normal amounts of food could easily turn into a grossly overweight condition; without his present amount of activity, the maintenance of desirable weight might require a daily intake of perhaps
1600 calories, just as we have observed in males who are relying on
caloric restriction to maintain their weights after low-calorie diets.

But there have been other tremendous payoffs in this particular
case. Six years ago this man's blood pressure was hard to control
with medication and he couldn't walk a block without resting. Today
his blood pressure is perfectly normal, and he can point to the
completion of two New York Marathons.

There is no way in the world that he would turn back the clock,
and live the way he used to.

However, when people have such strong genetic predispositions
to obesity, we should not deceive ourselves—it will take heroic
efforts in the way of physical activity to compensate and permit such
persons to approach the food intakes characteristic of average persons.

So, keep these examples in mind as I return to the question
posed in the first sentence of this chapter: What will it take to
manage *your* weight *without* a permanent change in eating habits?

Most people up to 75 pounds overweight can do it.

Our follow-up data in the Vanderbilt program show that people
who needed to lose 50 pounds or more when they first entered the
program several years ago, and who are now expending an extra
200 calories a day in physical activity, are averaging 47 pounds
lighter. That's the *activity* goal you reach in the fourth week of the
Metabolic Breakthrough Activity Program (you will not have lost 50
or more pounds in 4 weeks) and it verifies my statement that, on the
average, it takes about 200 calories a day in extra physical activity

to keep approximately 50 pounds of fat permanently off your body (if you have that much to lose).[1]

In a paper delivered at The Society for Behavioral Medicine, Stifler, Kaplan, and Lindewall reported that the average additional caloric expenditure in physical activity, usually walking, of women who had lost an average of about 60 pounds and men who had lost an average of about 75 pounds, and who were keeping it *all* off during the first year after a medically supervised low-calorie formula diet, was an extra *300 calories a day,* or about one hour of walking.[2]

I think that 45 minutes to 1 hour of extra activity can be fit into almost everyone's daily schedule. It is done most easily when you rely on walking or rebounding, which don't require a trip to a spa or special clothing. If you don't have an hour in one solid block of time, then you can always walk or bounce for any amount of time that happens to be convenient, several times a day. But, if weight control is truly a high priority, I don't see how you can avoid concluding that you owe an hour each day to yourself, for the sole purpose of weight control. You will soon discover that the benefits of activity go far beyond weight control: you will feel better, mentally and physically. In the final analysis, these benefits will keep you going.

So, the data indicate that for up to 50 pounds overweight, 45 minutes a day seems to work, and that 1 hour of brisk walking will do it for most people between 60 and 75 pounds overweight.

Setting Up Your Maintenance Program

If you have followed the Metabolic Breakthrough Plan to lose weight as I have indicated, maintenance is as "easy as pie."

Without realizing it, when you pursue the 28-Day Plan you are already including the basic ingredients in your new eating and activity habits. When you are ready to move into your permanent maintenance plan (or take time out from losing if you have a long way to go) just:

1. Continue with your activity program,
2. Make sure the AC portion of the AC/DC ratio is always at 8, and
3. That you continue to obtain adequate calcium and protein from the milk and meat groups of food—
THEN

4. Begin to add any food you like to your daily diet, one serving at a time, and get on your scale each day.

When your weight stabilizes (allowing for natural daily fluctuations of a pound or two) you will know how much you can eat without gaining, given your new activity level.

I want to emphasize that, when overweight is truly caused by eating more than a reasonable level of physical activity can burn off, most people find themselves in that condition because they eat too much fat or processed foods high in sugar, or both sugar and fat. In other words, the DC part of the AC/DC ratio climbs higher than 3 or 4, while the AC part falls below 8. NEVER add the third DC food until you have a total of 8 in the AC category. In fact, it is so hard to gain weight on AC foods that most reasonably active people can eat an almost unlimited quantity.

When you fill up first on the more healthful grains, fruits, and vegetables, your appetite for dense calories will be reduced—just remember, it takes six apples to equal the calories in one piece of apple pie. Have that piece of pie if you like—you are now active enough not to regain any weight when you do. But if you begin substituting a second, third, or fourth piece of pie for the fresh fruit you could have eaten instead, it's the concentration of fat and sugar in that dessert that can "outweigh" your new level of physical activity.

Would you like to know just how much you *will* be able to eat even before you get to maintenance?

It's quite easy to figure out if you are willing to take the time, but it does require some attention to the caloric value of foods, which you can look up in my quick Calorie Counter Lists on pages 136 to 149.

If you are a woman, presently eating between 1900 and 2000 calories per day, it is quite certain that you will be able to eat as much as you do today without regaining any weight. The same goes for men eating between 2400 and 2700 calories per day. It means about 45 minutes of Metabolic Breakthrough activities each day if you begin the program up to 50 pounds overweight, and about an hour a day if you are 75 pounds overweight. These activity levels can compensate for your present appetite and whatever metabolic predisposition to obesity you may have been born with.

You can verify these estimates as you approach your weight goal, just before setting up your maintenance plan, in the following way:

In the final weeks of your weight-loss program, every pound you lose contains about 3500 calories. (This is not true of the first week or two of the program, when you are still losing a considerable amount of water weight.) If you have been averaging a pound a week loss, you have been depleting your fat cells of about 500 calories a day (7 days × 500 calories = 3500 calories a week). It means you can add a regular-sized piece of pie and a glass of wine each day, if you choose, and not regain any weight. The long-term successful persons I have described in this chapter actually find that they can add somewhat more than this, and still not regain any weight, provided they continue to follow Metabolic Breakthrough Activity principles and keep their bodies programmed to burn these calories, not store them.

Set yourself a range of weight that is a permissible fluctuation— I suggest 3 to 5 pounds—and when you go over that, you know you have "outeaten" the limits of your activity program. You will have to cut back and, naturally, the place to cut is in the DC category.

Review my rules for eating slim in Chapter 5. Implementation of those rules, together with the level of activity you have reached at Week 4 of the activity program, is your assurance of permanent weight management.

The formula I have given you in the Metabolic Breakthrough Eating Plan and Activity Program would wipe out 99 percent of the obesity problem in the United States, once and for all. It will work for all but the most extreme metabolic abnormalities.

When you first begin the program, the most difficult part is *arranging your life* in order to put that formula into practice. Fortunately, it gets easier and easier as time goes on, rather than more and more difficult.

In the next section, I will give you some advice from the psychological perspective. Follow that advice and you will be confident of maintenance before you are ever put to the test.

PART V

The Psychology of
Successful Weight Management

23

GETTING YOUR HEAD ON STRAIGHT

This is a chapter filled with some tough talk.

You've seen the program. You've read the scientific evidence on which it is based. You know what it will take to make a Metabolic Breakthrough.

In a sense, you are in the position of a field marshal, girding your troops for battle. You know the enemy and the strategies required to conquer him.

The very first steps you take are really mental. The physical steps will follow—and follow and follow—if you are correctly prepared mentally.

From the psychological perspective, we need to get some things straight:

your attitude,

your expectations, and

your commitment.

With the correct attitude, realistic expectations, and complete commitment to the program, you *will* succeed. But, to continue the analogy, you must win the battle in a way that assures winning the peace that follows!

So let's be sure that you have a clear understanding of what it is going to take.

You must follow the 28-Day Metabolic Breakthrough Nutrition Plan and Activity Program *daily* to experience the Metabolic Breakthrough that I promise you.

Daily?

Yes, daily.

With respect to the Nutrition Plan, we are talking about just 28 days to maximize weight loss. If you have as much as 50 or 75 pounds to lose, and you want to lose it all without a break, then you must follow the AC/DC formula as your guide until you reach desired weight. When you reach your goal, for the sake of sound nutrition, you should continue to include at least eight servings of foods from the AC category before you indulge your appetite for DC foods.

However, my object is not to lock you into a way of eating that requires any more restraint than is absolutely necessary. We are surrounded with tasty, high-calorie foods. It is unreasonable to expect yourself to fight continually the perfectly normal biological urge to eat such foods when they are freely available. It is indeed rare that any overweight person develops a state of mind that makes it possible to *never again* indulge in tasty, high-calorie foods.

After you have made sure that your diet is basically nutritious, you want to have the ability to eat whatever you choose, at least in moderation. But you want to be absolutely certain that whatever you choose to eat is not going to start putting any of the weight you lost back on again.

Thus, for this very reason, we *are* talking about an *Activity Program* that must go on virtually every day *for life.* You can, of course, have a day off each week if you are tired, or if you were especially active the day before, or if you are just "under the weather."*

The key to permanent success lies in your commitment to physical activity.

With a correct attitude toward physical activity you will pursue it to the point where the payoff is so obvious and great that commitment will be automatic. But we have to get you there first.

From an attitudinal standpoint, you must appreciate that you cannot burn enough calories to eat without continual restraint nor can you change the fundamental metabolic processes that contribute to obesity with *occasional* physical activity.

Parking your car at the end of the lot when you visit the grocery store won't do it, nor will parking six blocks from your office.

Those three 20- or 30-minute workouts each week recommended by physical educators to increase cardiovascular endurance

*See page 65, where I discuss resting for one day.

won't do it, nor will two or three aerobic dance classes.

These are all steps in the right direction. They will contribute to your overall health, fitness, and feeling of well-being. They can and should be a *part* of your program.

But you cannot obtain significant *weight-related metabolic benefits* with such programs. You are simply deceiving yourself if you think that a little extra walking or a minimal, three times per week exercise schedule can burn enough calories to balance your *natural* appetite and caloric intake. That kind of an activity schedule doesn't balance mine and I don't think it will balance yours.

And, to be very honest about it, people who write diet and exercise books recommending such "easy-to-swallow" approaches know very well that exercise at that level cannot make a significant difference in weight management. They are afraid, however, that if they told you the *truth* it would scare you away and their programs would not be very popular! I prefer to tell you the truth as I see it, and help at least a few people, rather than be popular and help no one.

In addition to the frequency issue, occasional activity that fails to fulfill the guidelines of the Metabolic Breakthrough Plan cannot yield daily, round-the-clock alterations in your metabolic processes. That is, you cannot achieve a permanent change from a "fat" to a "thin" metabolism without daily activity at the level our bodies were bred to sustain during our evolutionary history, before our present state of technology.

You see, our bodies were designed to burn, in an average day, the energy required by at least 5 miles of walking, and probably something more like 7 or 8 miles. That's what it took for our ancestors to stay alive during the first few million years of our species' existence, right up until this century. Today, 99 percent of all energy expended in our society is done by machine.[1] Up until 100 years ago, from the start of the human race, it took several hundred calories more work each day just to get the job of living done: there were no cars and no electric labor-saving devices in our homes and offices. We walked a lot! And we flexed our muscles, men and women alike, a great deal more.

You must return to the level of ENERGY EXPENDITURE for which your body was NATURALLY DESIGNED if you want to EAT according to your NATURAL APPETITE.

I know that's a pretty stern lecture. But if you repeat it to yourself each day at the start of your program, you may be in for a surprise.

While a good deal of self-motivation and discipline are required to change your life-style in order to move your body around for that full 45 minutes each day that it takes to turn your system around, you are going to make an astonishing discovery:

Your feet were made for walking!

You have, buried in your genes, the ability to enjoy physical movement to the same extent that you enjoy good food or sex. All three *used to be* required for our existence, and nature has a way of building into our bodies a capacity to enjoy the things that are essential in order to ensure that we do them. Of course there has to be a balance between activity and rest, so we enjoy resting too. The value of a balance between activity and rest is easily seen in the fact that rest following physical activity is more complete and profound than rest following an inactive day, and that activity feels best, and we are best at it, when we are well rested.

But right now, there is a good chance activity doesn't feel as good to you as nature provided for only because you are rusty. You are out of condition for it. And you are carrying an unnecessary load of fat.

You will not fail to find some physical activity that is enjoyable if you approach the task in the same spirit with which you approach food and sex. If you don't like a particular recipe, you either throw it out or modify it to suit your taste. If you don't like sex one way, you do it another. Begin to explore various physical activities in exactly the same spirit and frame of mind and you will give your body a chance to express talents and experience pleasures that you probably never thought possible.

I have suggested walking and rebounding for starters and as fallback activities because they are the easiest and quickest ways to improve your metabolic processes and get yourself in shape for other things. You can, of course, use any combination of activities in which you can safely reach metabolic improvement intensity from the list given in Table 10-1, pp. 63–64.

So, get started.

You will soon be in shape to play the games you never thought you were capable of as an adult. In these you will rediscover the spirit of your childhood. Or perhaps you will want to dance and, like

Zorba, express your joy or chase your blues away. You may even end up climbing a mountain, or at least hiking a mountain trail. If you do that, you will get in touch with a primitive aspect of consciousness that also lies buried in your genes: as you wander through the forests or find it necessary to clamber over some difficult terrain, you will feel a kinship with your ancestors, and appreciate the strength and physical endurance that has kept the human race alive from its birth in a direct line to your very own existence.

A few months down the line I think you will find that the excitement in your thinner, more active future was worth the initial discipline and effort.

End of lecture.

24

A 10-SECOND TEST FOR MOTIVATION

"How can I maintain my motivation?"

This question never fails to come up in every group I lead and in every lecture that I give on weight management. It seems to be a puzzle and a problem to everyone, including the professionals. Volumes have been written on the general topic, and each year in the field of psychology entire symposia and conferences are devoted to it.

When it comes to weight control, however, there is no mystery to maintaining motivation. In spite of the stern tone of my last chapter, it's not a question of having to cultivate indomitable determination to fight forever against insurmountable odds. In fact, just thinking of the issue in that way—as a month after month, year after year (ugh!) problem—makes it hard to solve.

Motivation is only a matter of seconds. Indeed, whether you succeed in carrying out any task that is able to be done depends primarily on the actions you take in a very brief instant in time. I think I can prove this to you in the next few minutes.

First of all, I am sure that you have heard or read about the "laws of motion": how a body at rest tends to remain at rest until affected by some force, and, similarly, how a body moving in a particular direction tends to continue in that direction until it, too, is affected by some outside force.

Your body also tends to obey this law, at least in a meaningful figurative sense. We all, even the most active and physically fit people, occasionally feel reluctant to move, to take a planned walk or jog, or to start out for the dance class in which we have recently enrolled. We soon discover, however, that, if we can only point our toes toward the door and take the first steps out, the problem is solved.

Once we have swung into motion, the sluggishness disappears, whatever burdens we've been carrying seem to drop from our shoulders, and, in a way that almost defies analysis, we "feel free." It may take some effort and commitment to *get started*, but only *just enough to take the first steps*. When it comes to physical activity, once you get started the sensations begin to feel so good that it gets harder and harder to stop.

Here is a 10-Second Test for Motivation that will prove to you that motivation is only a matter of moments.

The 10-Second Test for Motivation

Pick a time when you have as little as 5 minutes (or as much as 45 minutes) at your disposal. I want you to take a walk, so consider it and make a decision to follow my directions. Make up your mind (we'll call this your initial commitment) to walk for at least 5 minutes.

Point your toes toward the door, step outside, and walk briskly for 10 seconds down the walkway (or corridor of your office building or whatever). That's about twenty steps worth of walking.

When you are twenty steps on your way, see if you can stop. It's just about impossible, especially when you think that fatness lies behind you and thinness in front! Do you really want to turn back now?

As you continue with your walk, consider what has happened and what you are doing. Can you see how, once you have made your commitment, what you do in just a matter of seconds sets the stage for successfully carrying out the entire action?

I know that you can pass this test, and, if you do, you will have succeeded in understanding the most crucial psychological issue involved in maintaining motivation. This is the psychological step that sets the stage for all the physiological changes that will automatically follow your movement through the 28-Day Program.

The best time to take this test is now. I know you have 5 minutes —just take a look at your watch. I know you have the time since you are reading this book. Stop reading and make a decision to walk for at least 5 minutes. It's more important than reading right now. Because you were not expecting this direction to take a walk, and have to make a conscious decision to do it, you will experience a perfect demonstration of the point I am trying to make. It means that you may have to overcome a certain amount of resistance, and assert your personal control over the laws of motion.

So get up and turn your feet in the direction of any open space. If you happen to be on an airplane, walk up and down the aisle! Then come back and read how maintaining your motivation for *anything* that is worthwhile doing in life is simply a matter of seconds.

I hope you finished the test and passed with flying colors. You had your own personal demonstration of the "laws of motion"—the problem of making the decision, maybe even the problem of *forcing* yourself to get up off your duff, and then the pleasant feeling of motion that makes it hard to stop. If for some reason you were not able to take the test right now (you were on a crowded subway or locked in a closet) take it as soon as possible.

If you take this test *every day* at precisely the time you have scheduled some physical activity, you will never be fat again.

You may find it easier to pass your daily test if you choose a social sport or set up appointments to walk with friends. And, no matter what happens in the outside world, you can always pass the test if you have a rebounder set up in a convenient spot. That is one of the reasons I suggest you buy one even if other physical activities, one of which you plan to do every day, are higher on your list of preferences. Rebounding is your fat-burning insurance policy, something you can fall back on when circumstances might prevent you from carrying out other forms of activity and make it easy to rationalize a failure to carry out your resolution.

After you have been passing this test each day for a certain period of time, you are going to learn something about yourself and about dealing with other aspects of your life. It's something that tends to happen to persons who engage in solo activities, such as walkers, joggers, and runners, more than to persons who engage in any other form of physical activity. It helps explain why persons who participate in such activities tend to show up in research on psychological characteristics as more *independent* and *self-confident* than persons who decide on any other kind of sport, as well as the average sedentary person.[1-3]

Changes occur at both conscious and unconscious levels.

At the conscious level you learn that even on the days when you are feeling tired or grouchy, and are almost absolutely certain that you don't feel like moving, going out for that walk or jog is only a matter of pointing your toes toward the door and taking the first step. You discover that, once you are on your way, the resistance to movement was a mirage—only a question of inertia. You were tired and sluggish simply because *you hadn't moved enough* to feel vigorous and inspirited.

When you feel tired or sluggish and you have not been physically active, you may have been overworked mentally or emotionally, but certainly not physically. Becoming physically active at just these times has an unexpected and especially large payoff. You are going to find that the worse you seem to feel, short of physical illness, the bigger the emotional lift you get from vigorous movement. At this point we don't know exactly why this occurs, but it does. It may have to do with certain hormones and chemicals in the central nervous system that influence our moods—the beta endorphins and catecholamines. Or it may result from the increased blood circulation, which supplies more oxygen to our brains. Or it may be just the change of scene, which relieves some overworked neural circuitry and stimulates a new train of thought. But physical activity when you feel most sluggish, aggravated, or reluctant acts like a waterfall washing the garbage out of your mind.

Going through the process of setting up your schedule to allow for physical activity and doing it every day has an additional impact that spreads unconsciously (if I weren't telling you about it) to other aspects of your life. You learn that, once you decide to do anything, the hardest job is usually getting started. Within moments after you begin any job to which you have assigned the priority "worth doing," the momentum of doing takes over. It operates just as surely as the initial inertia that seemed to stand in the way of beginning the job in the first place.

In setting up your schedule, you learn that you have the right to have at least 45 minutes of your very own each day in the pursuit of your own health and happiness. Furthermore, when you assert

302 / The Psychology of Successful Weight Management

that right, others will respect it. And they come to respect *you*, too, as a person strong enough to take on the responsibility for your own well-being. Perhaps this is what leads to the increased self-confidence and self-esteem that shows up in the psychological tests of walkers and runners.

So, set up your schedule for physical activity and think of your first twenty steps as your Daily 10-Second Test for Motivation. It's a simple test to pass. Maintaining your motivation presents no problem when you think of it as I suggest: it takes but a few moments to overcome your inertia and then you can let your momentum carry you through to the finish.

You may find it harder to stop than to begin.

25

THE ENVIRONMENT FOR SUCCESS

It's not your fault you're fat.

Until today.

I mean by this that hereditary factors may have been operating to make it easier for you to store more fat than the average person. Or, if you are overweight because you eat too much or exercise too little, you acquired these patterns of behavior according to the same principles of learning that determined whether you speak English or Chinese. No one blames you for learning to speak your native tongue, and you can't be blamed for learning the eating and activity habits that are encouraged in your environment.

However, you *can* learn to speak another language. That's up to you. It all depends upon whether you are willing to take the initiative. The same goes for getting slim and staying that way.

To learn a new language you have to put aside the time, and you have to study and practice. If you don't, your brain won't make the necessary physiological changes that represent "knowing the language." No study and no practice equal no learning.

And once you know the language, if you don't keep using it, it will tend to slip way from you.

The same goes for your weight. You now know the real issues in weight control and what it's going to take to be slim. You have to make the physiological changes that will get you down to desired weight in a way that ensures permanent success. You are going to have to put aside the time to be active—and do it. And you will have to stay active, or your control will slip away from you. You have to keep moving your body, or, just as with your knowledge of a foreign language, if you don't use it, you'll lose it.

In most cases, people are overweight because of a combination of factors: there is some hereditary predisposition interacting with fat eating habits and a lack of activity. The environment plays a major role in determining whether you eat in a way that encourages obesity, and whether it is easy to be sedentary or active.

Few people are aware of the power that the environment has over their behavior. Each year I see some striking illustrations of this power in the behavior and weight changes among the students I teach in my classes at Vanderbilt. A weight gain in their first year away from home is so common among the girls that it has come to be called "The Freshman 15." I am not sure that the girls actually do average a gain of 15 pounds their first year, but that is how they refer to it.

Each year I do a survey among the students, looking at the changes that take place in diet and activity that occur as a result of entering a college environment. Between 95 and 98 percent of the students indicate changes in their pattern of eating and activity as a result of entering or returning to the college environment after being away for the summer. There is a significant increase in high-fat and processed foods, and a significant decrease in physical activity.

What about you? Take a minute to think about yourself and how "circumstances" affect your behavior: what happens to you if you take a vacation, go to a wedding or cocktail party, or expose yourself to a buffet? How about those business trips, or changing jobs?

If you made a resolution to become active in the past and ultimately failed to follow through, what happened to get in the way of your resolution? I think you will see that there were strong environmental forces operating to make something other than activity seem more necessary or more rewarding. In addition, you may not have known how to deal with motivation and the laws of motion I discussed in the previous chapter. If you don't know how to deal with your inertia, it is easy for the pleasures of the kitchen or couch to win out over the pleasures of the open road.

Human existence involves continual interaction with the environment. We really deal with a number of different environments each day, and we have well-learned patterns of behavior for each of them, from our bedrooms and kitchens to our offices and the grocery store.

But we also have tremendous power *to alter* our environments. Once we alter them by taking the initiative and changing their characteristics, we begin to respond to a whole new set of environmental influences.

You can do a great deal to make weight management easier if you take the initiative and make a few changes in your environment. Once the changes have been made, you don't have to do conscious battle against the old forces that were preserving your fat eating and activity patterns. Sometimes a few key changes in your environment take only minutes to make, but, once you make them, they continue to support a lifetime of successful weight management without further effort.

Setting Up Your Active Environment

If you are going to be active—walking more, playing some active game, or participating in some exercise or dance class—virtually every day for the rest of your life, what are you going to need to change in order to accomplish this?

Let me tell you first about my own experiences.

My own transition from being a very sedentary person to becoming a relatively active one offers a good example of the comparative ease with which a man can change his life-style and find that the world around him is ready to collaborate. In fact, it was a real eye-opener to contrast my situation (and that of most males) with the problems women face. I'll get to that in a moment.

I remember just as though it were yesterday the very first afternoon after I decided to lose weight and get active over 20 years ago, when I called my wife on the phone and said, "Hi, honey—I've got a tennis match after I finish work today at five. I'll be home about seven, so go ahead and feed the kids, I'll eat whatever's left." I don't even recall if I volunteered to clean up or help get the children ready for bed, but I do recall her answer. It was a simple "That's fine. I'll see you then. Have a good game." And mind you, my wife has always been a working woman, with a schedule as busy as mine, and sometimes even busier. She was, of course, just as eager as I was for me to lose weight and get fit because of my health problems.

So tennis went down first on my daily schedule, and everything else got worked in around it.

Physical activity is *always* down first on my daily schedule. Sometimes it is not so easy to work out. During the rat study I described previously, I often had to get to the lab by 7:30 A.M. I like to run in the afternoons during the week, but the temperature was in the nineties everyday for a long period and I had a number of late afternoon meetings. I began going to bed at 9 and getting up at 5, instead of 6, so that I could run for an hour before work. It is very nice to watch the sun come up.

I do a great deal of traveling, to meetings or to give lectures and participate in workshops. When I know that taking the time for an hour's jog will be impossible during a full day of travel, I schedule that day for my day off.* Usually, however, there is a group of runners participating in whatever meeting I'm going to, and the organizers of most professional meetings have taken to scheduling times for running (or walking) these days. There are so many of us now.

But it wasn't always that way. I used to do site visits to evaluate programs for the government or for different professional organizations when physical activity was not as great a part of the life-style among physicians and psychologists as it is today. Meetings might start with a 7 A.M. breakfast and continue, with only meal breaks, until 10 P.M. I began to call my hosts at the program I was about to visit and the other members of my site visit team to request that the meeting be scheduled around a two-hour break for physical activity at some point during the day. Fifteen years ago that elicited a great deal of surprise, but never any resistance. Everyone knew they ought to take a break, but they thought they were the only ones that wanted or needed it.

We got just as much work done as ever, and felt much better doing it.

Most men, no matter what their line of work, can usually schedule physical activity into their daily lives with very little difficulty once they decide it's more important than *just one thing* that now takes 45 minutes.

It's often a different story for a working woman. When women

*See page 65, where I discuss resting for one day.

decide to pursue a career outside the home, *they as well as their mates* assume that they are still going to be full-time mothers and house-wives the moment the "working day" is over. Even in more egalitarian families, it is very rare that working husbands assume a full share of the family's household and child-rearing responsibilities.

This is gradually changing. If you are a woman about to begin your weight management program, and you have a husband who believes in taking on his full share of the family duties (and carries through), you should have little problem getting collaboration to find 45 minutes a day for physical activity. You have only to decide where your priorities lie, and eliminate 45 minutes of whatever you are doing now that is not as high on the list as getting slim and staying that way.

You are the only one standing in your way.

And just a word about babies:

If you are a new mother, it is probably most important that you be as physically active as is possible after your baby is born if you want to control your weight and reestablish your pre-pregnancy balance of hormones. Being pregnant turns on fat-storage mechanisms, and it's time to turn them off now that the baby is born. You do it better by staying active. Check with your physician and get his recommendations.

It's up to you to take the initiative and set up your husband's role in child care if he doesn't do it as a matter of course. Forty-five minutes a day being a father isn't a lot to ask even if your husband is not the fully sharing type, or even if you don't expect or want him to be.

Determination and negotiation—that's the name of the game.

Here are more examples:

Phyllis, whom I mentioned back in Chapter 7, has two teenage children living at home and works from 8 to 5. She gets up early enough to meet a group of walking friends for a two-mile walk before work. She does the same after work. If she didn't, she wouldn't be on her feet long enough to burn the 1950 calories she eats every day and continue to keep that 45 pounds of fat off. And, by the way, her children learned quite quickly how to get themselves off to school in the morning without her help.

Barbara, a schoolteacher, has two young children of her own that need supervision to get ready for school and their lunches made. What with taking care of the family, teaching, and preparing for classes, she never thought she could organize her day for consistent physical activity. So, she put the problem to her husband for solution. Her husband took over the early morning family responsibilities, and Barbara now has 45 minutes for a walk before work.

Jenny found three other women at work who also wanted to lose weight. They organized themselves into the "walk for lunch bunch" and get half an hour in every day. (They don't sit around for coffee breaks anymore, either.)

I could give you many more examples, but I think you get the point.

If you need social support and walking companions, start thinking of ways to get it. You know many others who need to lose weight and get fit, as well as yourself. And you have neighbors. If you can't step into an ongoing group of active people, get it going yourself.

Engineering a Healthy Eating Environment

Most persons up to 50 pounds overweight will be able to eat pretty much according to their natural appetites when they reach the fat-burning activity goal of the Metabolic Breakthrough Plan. Some people will want to make a change for the better in the nature of their diets even if they can eat as many high-calorie foods as they like. Others will be able to "outeat" any moderate level of activity and must find a way to control their appetite for (I'll say it) junk foods.

Because the most important dietary change you can make is to see that your AC/DC ratio is always at 8/2, or that you always eat those eight servings of whole grains, fruits, and vegetables before you indulge yourself on candy, cake, and cookies, *what changes in your kitchen, shopping habits, and food preparation are you going to make in order to accomplish this?*

Suppose, just like myself, you normally eat in a nutritious manner and you are fairly active, but you know that you can't forever and always resist your favorite kinds of cookies, cakes, or confections if they are *always* right in front of your nose?

What are you willing to do to remove these temptations?

Here is another personal story that illustrates the point I want to make.

I just gained 4 pounds.

The explanation is rather simple.

I have a great appreciation for chocolate chip cookies, chocolate candy, sugar/cream-filled cookies, etc. In spite of my high level of activity I will begin to gain weight if I have these foods in my kitchen on a continual basis. I may not eat any of them for days on end, but if they are there, day after day, week after week, I'll finally get around to them.

Wouldn't you?

And, by the way, freezing doesn't help to keep me away from cookies, doughnuts, and cakes. I discovered long ago that they taste great frozen.

During the 108 days in which I was fattening the rats in the research study I described earlier, the most convenient place to store the high-fat, high-sugar foods was in my kitchen near my food processor. There they were and my whole family would binge on occasion. Three out of four of us gained weight.

That particular study is over. The food is gone. We have all returned to our former weights.

Take a look at your own kitchen and your own pantry. Do you store a nice variety of DC foods? If you do, will you stick to your Nutrition Plan for the number of days it will take to reach your desired weight?

Can you have such food around and not overeat to the point where your new activity level will burn the calories off?

If I have such foods freely available, I know that I cannot succeed in ignoring them forever.

Twenty years ago, long before the behaviorists invented their long list of strategies to help modify eating habits, I knew exactly what I needed to do if I was going to lose 70-plus pounds in any reasonable length of time.

I created my own periodic, artificial famines.

With my wife's collaboration, we simply got these high-calorie foods completely out of the house for three to four weeks at a time. After that, we would buy pastry goods, candy, or ice cream on special occasions—*exactly enough for a dinner party or for one or two servings for each member of the family.* Up until my rat study, we never had a constant supply of candy, desserts, and processed snack foods around the house, and I never gained weight, except for my normal and temporary daily fluctuations.

Although I need approximately 3000 calories a day to maintain my weight, and although I eat large quantities of fruit, fresh and dried, to keep a high ratio of complex carbohydrates in my diet, I proved once again during this recent study that I can always find room for a couple of candy bars after a complete meal—even when I feel full.

You may find that you can develop a strategy to ignore DC foods around the house in order to implement your nutrition plan. If you can, great. The behaviorists have suggested special wrappings, using labels on the packaging with the names of other family members pasted on them, and special, out-of-sight storage areas (this works for me *for short periods*). That may be all that's necessary for you.

If these strategies will not work for you, you'd better have a friendly meeting with your housemates and create an artificial famine for an agreed-upon period of time. Why not 28 days as a starter if you have more than 15 pounds to lose?

Here is a very helpful tip for people who have a real yen for sweets and who, no matter how hard they try to restrain themselves or to substitute artificial sweeteners for sugar *most* of the time, still end up overeating on candy, cakes, and other sweets more frequently than they like. While it is *not an essential part of the program*, it has helped many people who feel "addicted" to sweets. This advice also works for people who feel that they use too much salt for the good of their health.

If you quit eating highly sweetened (or salty) foods for a few weeks you may make an interesting discovery. Taste sensitivity to such flavors appears to increase when they are removed from the diet for any length of time. In order to increase your sensitivity to sweetness and saltiness, so that you will require less to satisfy your taste in the future, you must remove sugar and salt from your diet for at least one week or, better, two. If you have a real yen for sweet or salty flavors, this is well worth doing.

You must give up the diet drinks and all foods with artificial sweeteners as well.

Artificial sweeteners only keep your sweet tooth alive, perhaps at a heightened level. They don't fool your body, which knows quite quickly that they are not providing any nutritional value, and there is some evidence that artificial sweeteners may actually turn on food-seeking behavior. In other words, artificial sweeteners do not appear to help a bit in weight management.

So, if you will stop using salt, sugar, and artificial sweeteners for a week or two, you are almost certain to find that it takes less to satisfy your palate should you decide to add them back to your diet.

But a word of warning from a person who knows: if you are at all like me, you will gradually begin to eat more and more sweetened desserts and salty snacks all over again if you return to keeping a constant supply of them around the house.

I never will again. When I begin my next study that requires fattening rats, I will get someone else to store the food who doesn't have the same appetite for it that I do.

When it comes to making changes in the environment to help support new eating habits, men usually have a much easier time of it than do women. When a man comes home to his family, declares his desire to lose weight, and says to his wife, "Honey, I really love your apple pie and chocolate cake, but let's not have any this month, until I get this weight off," he usually gets full collaboration.

But let a woman announce her desire to do the same—not bake or purchase such foods for any length of time—and she is likely to be greeted with, "You mean I have to go on a diet because you are trying to lose weight?" Women are supposed to have whatever willpower it takes to pass up these foods while all the other members of the family are eating to their hearts' content.

Perhaps you think the other family members shouldn't be denied their desserts and snack foods. You have growing young ones active in school sports, and a skinny mate. In this case you should first reconsider whether you are doing anyone, including them, a favor by having such food around *if they are not eating nutritiously* to begin with.

If other members of your family aim first for the highly processed, high-fat and high-sugar foods, and are not getting those eight servings of AC foods each day because they "don't like" fruits and vegetables, you are not doing them any favor by satisfying their demands. As I have already explained, humans have a preference for sweetness combined with fat and salt, but we don't have a built-in discriminating function that tells us which sweet foods are healthiest. In addition, we don't have a turn-off mechanism that tells us "enough" when our preferred flavors are combined with a higher concentration of calories than occurs in their natural form. Our predispositions for flavor can be exploited by food processors, and they *are* being exploited. But not for *your* profit.

Perhaps you don't wish to fight it out with your family. The tensions would be too great.

You are not alone. While men almost always find no opposition, a large percentage of women do. The family situation can get unbearable if Dad is denied his dessert or the kids their candy and snack foods for even a week or two.

This puts you face to face with the ultimate reality. It's there even in the most favorable situations, when everyone tries to help. You must face it whenever "something happens" and you outeat the amount of calories your level of activity can burn:

Weight control is your responsibility.

It's not your mate's, your family's, your doctor's, or your friends'.

If you can't or don't wish to change a fat eating environment, you have no choice left.

You must remove *yourself* from the environment that threatens you.

And just as what you do in a few moments of time determines whether you carry out your daily intention to be active, so do a few brief moments determine what will happen to your Nutrition Plan during the period of weight loss or at times that you might outeat your activity level.

When you are faced with a temptation that doesn't fit your plan, get yourself away immediately—the next room, out of doors, into the basement, or hide in a bathroom!

Move fast, and have other activities set up so that engaging in them is easy the moment you take the first step.

If you can't sit and stare at the goodies while others are eating, or if you can't be satisfied with the fruit and cheese you may have planned for your own dessert, or if you will eat the fruit and cheese first and *then* get into the pie and cake when you finish—GET OUT!

If you choose any other course of action, you are simply letting the unconscious power of those two million years of evolution, which says "eat, eat" in every cell of your body, take over. No amount of willpower based on your desire to look or feel better can win out forever if you try to prolong this uneven battle.

Only a disappearing act has any hope of working, together with the substitution of some other rewarding activity.

Now it's up to you to make your choice.

PART VI

The Great Escape,
or
Are You a Refugee from a Low-Calorie Diet?

26

COPING WITH THE FAILED
LOW-CALORIE DIET

Because of the powerful advertising campaigns, and the apparent quick and easy success, several million people in the United States have been on diets of 800 or fewer calories during the past two years.

If you are one of the vast majority of persons who tried one of these diets but failed to reach your desired weight, I know you are experiencing a mixture of pleasure with your partial success together with some frustration over your failure to make it all the way.

I also know the reluctance you experience every time you consider going back on that same diet in order to continue to lose weight. If you are like most people I have interviewed when they are about to enter our program, your whole body seems to revolt at the thought of starting all over again on the last diet you used. The deprivation you experienced and your relative lack of success don't leave a very good taste in your mouth! And, for the great majority of people, no diet seems to work as well the second time around. Perhaps that is why people are always looking for a *new* diet.

Why Diets Don't Work as Well the Second Time Around

There are several reasons why no low-calorie diet works as well the second time around. The psychological aspects are intertwined with the physiological.

Having read this far, you know that, when you finish a low-calorie diet, your metabolism has slowed to the point where you need only a fraction of your pre-diet requirement to keep yourself going. In addition, the hormones and enzymes that promote fat storage increased in activity the moment you increased your food intake. They may remain elevated in activity until you regain all of the weight you have lost. Because you probably don't need as many calories to maintain your present weight as you did before you began your original diet, when you begin again for the second time (or third, or fourth, etc.) weight loss simply cannot proceed at the same rate that it did the first time.

So there you are, dieting just as severely as ever, but not losing weight as fast as you did the first time. Is it any wonder a person feels discouraged? Motivation to continue under these conditions is sure to evaporate even faster than it did the first time around.

Perhaps in the past you felt guilty or ashamed of your inability to stick with a diet that some expert, or some flashy advertising, claimed would be so easy. I certainly hope you realize that there is no need to blame yourself: your frustration, discouragement, and reluctance to proceed are really rooted in biological reality. It isn't only your conscious brain that is resisting the diet—it's every single cell in your body.

In order to start losing weight efficiently once again after you have gotten only part of the way to desired weight on a low-calorie diet, you must reverse the slowdown in your metabolic processes and counter the heightened activity of those fat-storing hormones and enzymes that are working so hard to prevent you from continuing to lose weight.

How to Succeed with the 28-Day Metabolic Breakthrough Plan after a Recent Low-Calorie Diet

To start losing weight once again, you must do everything you can to speed up metabolic processes. You must turn *ON* fat-burning mechanisms and turn *OFF* the fat-storage mechanisms that have become so active.

You can use the 28-Day Metabolic Breakthrough Plan with these special modifications to speed the process:

Step 1. Begin immediately to implement the Nutrition Plan and Activity Program outlined on pages 89–135.

Step 2. Because you have already lost some weight, you may be in condition to use the Advanced Metabolic Break-through Activity Program and reach the fat-burning goal of Week 4 somewhat earlier, but don't overdo. Instead, maximize your fat burning by using Super Booster principles: moderate activity after meals, or activity at Metabolic Breakthrough Intensity before dinner. Because of your adaptive metabolic slowdown, *you may not start to lose weight until you have worked up to the fat-burning goal of Week 4.* Be patient with your body until you can turn your slowed metabolism around.

Step 3. Weigh yourself daily. By the time you have followed the *Week 4* Metabolic Breakthrough Activity Program for a full week you may have countered your metabolic slow-down and your increased fat-storage potential. This may be all that it takes. In this case, weight loss will begin again at about 1 to 3 pounds a week. However, I must warn you that, if you are only recently off a low-calorie diet, it may take several weeks for your body to readjust and for weight loss to start again at that rate.

Step 4. If, and only if, your weight loss does not reach a minimum of 1 pound a week, make the following modifications in the 28-Day Metabolic Breakthrough Nutrition Plan:

a. Cut out the second DC allowance. This will lead to an AC/DC ratio of 8/1. *Of all nutrients, fat is most easily incorporated into your fat cells.* If you have difficulty losing weight, you must take away the nutrient (fat) that your hormones and enzymes have learned to store in your fat cells. Remember, this step is temporary. Once you reach goal weight, you will be able to include more DC foods in your diet.

b. Replace low-fat milk products with skim milk products.

c. If you don't start to lose weight, cut out one or two grain servings for up to 28 days. This will reduce your AC/DC ratio to as low as 6/1 on a temporary basis. Your calories will be down to about 1000 (for a woman; about 1500 to 1600 for a man). After 28 days, the Metabolic Breakthrough Activity Program should have brought about some significant changes in your fat-burning potential and you should restore those grain servings.

Steps 4a, 4b, and 4c are *temporary* steps to facilitate weight loss in difficult cases. A sample Daily Nutrition Plan and Activity Program that you may follow for a maximum of 4 weeks is presented on page 320. Compare that plan with the regular forms on pages 104 to 135 and you will see that all you need to do to follow the program is to remove up to two grain servings (along with all but one DC allowance) and meet a daily AC/DC ratio of 6/1.

I suggest that, each day while you are eating this small amount of food, you take a multiple vitamin and mineral capsule containing the RDAs of all the essential vitamins and minerals.

If you are one of those persons who is convinced that you cannot lose weight on anything but a starvation diet, you *must* follow the recommendations I have just made exactly. Change the Eating Record forms in the 28-Day Plan (pp. 104–35) to conform to these specifications, that is, one DC allowance and a daily AC/DC ratio of 6/1.

Keep in mind that the key to a Metabolic Breakthrough lies in reaching 45 minutes of whole-body movement at Metabolic Breakthrough Intensity every day.

After 28 days on the reduced Nutrition Plan, add back those grain servings and return to the regular program. You may find that you can continue to lose with a higher caloric intake because of the metabolic improvements brought about by physical activity. When you reach goal weight, follow my general suggestions in Chapter 22 for setting up your maintenance plan and examine the suggestions I make in the next chapter for people who are going directly into maintenance from a low-calorie diet.

If you cannot lose weight satisfactorily by following the Metabolic Breakthrough Plan with the above modifications, there is every reason to believe that you are the victim of at least some minor metabolic or hormone abnormality that may require knowledgeable *and sympathetic* medical attention.

Take your completed 28-day record to your physician and discuss your weight problem *with these data in front of him.*

But remember, the program must be followed exactly for a minimum of 28 days in order to illustrate conclusively that your system is not responding to a healthy and reasonable weight management regimen.

In all of my years as director of the Vanderbilt Weight Management Program, I have found it necessary to reduce calories to 800 per day in only *two* cases in order to achieve satisfactory weight loss. In both instances these were women in their fifties with a lifelong history of overweight and continual dieting. And no male has ever needed to go below 1800 (unless he has done so without my knowledge). The only times we ever use low-calorie intakes are for research purposes.

The Metabolic Breakthrough Plan will work for over 99 percent of all overweight people. But, as I have just indicated, I also know that there are indeed a few women who must, because of physiological abnormalities, reduce their caloric intake to an extremely low level in order to lose weight. And there are also some people who, for health reasons or the need for surgery, must reduce rather quickly. In my opinion, low-calorie dieting should be done under professional supervision.

And please heed my final words of advice:

Do not go on any low-calorie diet that weakens you, makes you feel listless and lethargic, and does not supply the energy you need to pursue the Metabolic Breakthrough Activity Program at the same time.

It may be just that kind of severe dieting, in which you have failed to take the steps that can counter the inevitable metabolic slowdown and post-dieting biochemical changes, that has created your difficult condition in the first place. *There is no sense in making a bad situation worse!*

Sample Nutrition Plan and Activity Program to Facilitate Weight Loss in Difficult Cases

ACTIVITY PROGRAM

45 Minutes per Day at Metabolic Breakthrough Intensity

NUTRITION PLAN

	RECOMMENDED SERVINGS
Milk group (skim milk products)	2
Meat group	2
AC group	
Grains	2
Fruits	2
Vegetables	2
DC group	
Fat	1
AC/DC Ratio must equal 6/1	

27

EATING NORMALLY AFTER A LOW-CALORIE DIET

If you have just finished losing weight on a low-calorie diet and if you have made it all the way to your desired weight, you deserve, first of all, a real pat on the back. You have won your first battle, and I hope that whatever maintenance plan you are using it's been working. I hope that you are reading this chapter before regaining a single one of your hard-lost pounds.

However, if you are a sedentary person and have been on a diet of 800 or fewer calories in the recent past, you have probably found that you cannot eat more than about 1200 calories a day (if you are a woman) without regaining weight. And, if you are a man, chances are that you cannot eat more than 1800 calories without gaining. As I discussed in Chapter 22, these are the typical maintenance levels that seem to be required after completing a low-calorie diet. Since very few people are able to stick with such low intakes when there are so many tempting high-calorie foods available, maintenance plans that are so low in calories have very little chance of succeeding over a long period of time.

For this reason, I want to show you how to apply Metabolic Breakthrough principles, still keep that weight off, and begin to eat once more like a *normal* person.

My goal is to show you how to eat *at least 400 to 600 calories more per day than you can at the present time* and still maintain desirable weight.

I believe it is very important that you cultivate an ability to do this. It is extremely difficult to obtain adequate nutrition over a long period of time on fewer than 1600 to 1800 calories. Vitamin and mineral supplementation cannot assure the level or kind of nutrition human beings were meant to obtain from the wide variety of foods that occur naturally. Modern nutritional science does not yet have the knowledge to fabricate a standard artificial formula that can be put into a pill or powder which will satisfy everyone's nutritional requirements over the long haul. The very best standard formula will be unbalanced and inadequate for some people and it may lack trace elements. You may get too much or too little of some nutrients, and this can change your need for others. In addition, your diet is likely to be rather low in fiber. If you have experienced any uncomfortable change in your intestinal functions while on a low-calorie diet, then you are already aware of one of the more obvious problems. When your system goes out of whack, it's telling you that what you're doing is probably not good for you!

It is worth reemphasizing that your best assurance for good health and adequate nutrition lies in your ability to eat *plenty* of a wide variety of healthful foods—*without gaining weight!*

And you will be able to do just that by following the 28-Day Metabolic Breakthrough Plan with the special adaptations that are required to boost your metabolism after a low-calorie diet.

However, I must warn you that a return to normal intake without significant weight gain may require a transition period of several weeks or even more. Having been on a low-calorie diet, you may already have discovered this for yourself. In the case of one woman volunteer who used a 600-calorie diet to lose 65 pounds in 19 weeks in one of our research projects, it took 14 weeks to build back to 1800 calories in spite of her having averaged at least 45 minutes of daily walking throughout the weight-loss period and during the transition back to a stable maintenance plan. When she upped her intake only 200 calories per day, from 600 to 800, she gained 3 pounds during the first week due to the rehydration effect that I will explain in a moment. The gain was temporary, as it is likely to be in your case as well should it occur when you follow these directions.

How to Increase Your Food Intake
without Gaining Weight

It is essential to add calories to your diet *very slowly* when you begin to change from your present low-calorie maintenance plan to the higher intake that you will find possible on the Metabolic Breakthrough Plan. You must be cautious and adhere to certain dietary principles for several reasons:

1. When you increase food intake after a low-calorie diet your body is subject to what is called a "rehydration effect." This means a very rapid accumulation of water, *often above normal levels,* which shows up on your scale as a very rapid and discouraging weight gain. It takes place because of

a. the increased sodium that naturally occurs in a larger quantity of food,

b. an increased speed in the rebuilding of any muscle mass that was lost during the low-calorie diet (muscle tissue is 75 to 80 percent water),

c. rebuilding of lost energy stores in the form of glycogen (another 75 to 80 percent water in solution with this sugar), and

d. increased water production from the metabolism of more food.

2. Certain foods are more likely to lead to weight gain than are others. If you restore foods that are high in sodium, you will experience an unnecessary amount of water retention. Even adding healthful complex carbohydrates can do this to a certain extent. The real danger, however, lies in foods high in fat and low in fiber. It's these foods from my DC list that will be most easily converted to fat storage. They should be avoided during the first part of your transition if you want to guarantee your success.

The Four-Step Transitional Metabolic Breakthrough Plan

Follow this Four-Step Plan to make a transition from your present maintenance program to the Metabolic Breakthrough Plan:

Step 1. Begin immediately with the 28-Day Metabolic Breakthrough Nutrition Plan and Activity Program on pages 89–135. For most people, the caloric intake on their present maintenance plan will be approximately equal to the Breakthrough Nutrition Plan. This is temporary, of course—our goal is to increase your potential by several hundred calories.

Step 2. Since you have already reached desired weight, you should find it possible to use the Advanced Activity Program and reach the fat-burning goal of Week 4 somewhat earlier, *but do not overdo.* To maximize metabolic improvement, consider scheduling your activity before dinner whenever possible, if only during the first few weeks during this transition.

Step 3. Weigh yourself daily. You may begin to lose weight in Week 2 or 3 because of the increased caloric expenditure and fat burning ability that occurs as a result of the Metabolic Breakthrough Activity Program. Allow this to occur for 1 week to be sure it is not a question of water loss. A weight gain is also possible if you perspire a great deal during your Activity Program. Many people overshoot the mark in their fluid intake when they get active, especially in hot weather. Do not be concerned. It is natural. Change nothing and your system will adjust. The *more* fluid you drink, the faster it will adjust, so be sure to have at least eight glasses of water a day.

Step 4. When you reach the activity goal of the Metabolic Breakthrough Program (or if you have started to lose weight before reaching that goal), begin to add certain foods, *and only the foods that I will now suggest,* in the amounts I suggest, until you find that your weight has stabilized. Then you can begin to deviate according to your natural appetite without regaining any weight.

Adding to Your Nutrition Plan

A. Add *one serving of a fruit or vegetable high in fiber* to the regular Metabolic Breakthrough Nutrition Plan. Refer to the AC List on pp. 141–42, or to Fruit and Vegetable List I on pages 140 to 142, for your selection. The next day, if you show no weight gain, continue with the next addition. Otherwise, stick with this fruit or vegetable addition until you stabilize.

B. Now add one more serving (about 3 ounces more) of a high-protein food from the meat group or another serving of a low-fat food from the milk group. Continue to monitor your weight and make no further additions until you stabilize.

C. Now add another serving of food from the AC group. You will now be weight stable with an added protein serving, and two additional selections from the AC group. This will give you an AC/DC ratio of 10/1, or 10/2 if you have used the second DC allowance. Stick with this until you have determined that you are stable at that intake.

D. It is a good idea to avoid all foods high in sodium content while you are making this transition.*

And now comes the fun. Once you have reached your activity goal, increased your intake by the 300 or so calories according to the above nutrition plan, and found that your weight is stable, it is perfectly okay to start indulging yourself a bit. There is room for extra DC foods occasionally, quite possibly even three allowances each day. But you must maintain your Metabolic Breakthrough Activity Program, and, as you begin to add foods in the DC category, your daily nutrition plan must still include those eight servings of AC foods to ensure the high fiber intake that can waste some of those tasty high-fat calories.

I know that all of these directions can seem like a lot of bother, but they form a program that does work, even in very difficult instances, such as the transition from the 600-calorie diet I described earlier.

There is another way to make the transition that does not quite have the guarantees that go with the careful program I have just outlined. You can simply participate in the Metabolic Breakthrough Activity Program, which will turn off the fat-conserving processes that were encouraged by your low-calorie diet, and play it by ear with your nutrition plan. Watch your weight each day, and adjust your present maintenance approach as needed. However, this is not as likely to succeed if your diet is high in fat and low in fiber, for the various reasons I have discussed throughout this book.

*A list of foods high in sodium appears on page 149.

EPILOGUE

This short epilogue is an absolute pleasure to write, and I know it is going to be an even greater pleasure for you to live.

I don't have to give you a "Lifetime Maintenance" DIET!

You will soon be done with calorie counting, food exchange lists, diet group meetings, and guilt over the bad eating habits you never really had.

Happy walking, bouncing, and *eating!*

APPENDIX A

HOW MUCH SHOULD YOU WEIGH?

A rather large number of Tables of Desirable Weights have been published, some based on research findings and others for use by commercial weight-control programs. Differences among them may have confused you.

The differences are due to the fact that most research has sought to determine the weight, for age, sex, and height, that has the best relationship to longevity—that is, what weight is correlated with long life.

The weight-control program charts tend to suggest higher weights because they take into consideration that persons coming into these programs are at least somewhat predisposed to obesity. It may be unreasonable to expect persons who are by nature heavier to weigh as little as the Desirable Weights Charts suggest. Desirable weight in many of the research studies proved to be about 10 percent below the average weight of the population. And I agree that that is an unreasonable expectation for persons who naturally tend to be on the heavier side—in fact, for such persons, desirable weight, at 10 percent below average, might prove to be quite unhealthy. However, I know of no research that examines this issue.

In my view, desirable weight is an individual matter that cannot be adequately handled by statistics alone. *Your* desirable weight must take into account both physical and psychological factors on a personal basis.

But let's take a look at the statistics first.

Most leading health authorities are now of the opinion that there is no clear-cut relationship between weight and a shortened life span for people less than 20 or 25 percent over *average* weight.* This means that it has been impossible to find a direct correlation between overweight—up to about 20 percent—and a shorter life span, *as long as that degree of overweight is not also associated with some health problem, such as hypertension or diabetes, which does appear to shorten life.* Thus, as long as you remain in good health, a small degree of overweight does not decrease the probability that you will live as long as your thinner friends (and 20 percent is the cutoff point that most authorities use to define obesity).

The problem with being overweight is that many illness *are* associated with that extra weight. For example, on the average, blood pressure will be 6 to 8 mm higher for each 10 percent above average weight. The likelihood of adult onset diabetes also increases. In other words, if you can avoid the illness associated with obesity, the *mortality* rate does not appear to increase until persons reach more than 20 percent above average weight. But the *morbidity* rate—that is, the likelihood of certain illness—does increase with increasing obesity. The list of obesity-related illnesses and symptoms includes:

hypertension
high blood lipid levels
impaired glucose tolerance
high uric acid levels and gout
adult onset (Type II) diabetes
pulmonary dysfunction
physical performance incapacities (such as an
      arthritic problem aggravated by obesity) and
      difficulties in locomotion, balance, or posture
      (which make some overweight persons prone to accidents)

Many of these illness are partially or wholly reversible with weight loss, which is how we know that obesity may be related to causality. Naturally, if you suffer form any of these obesity-related problems, it is usually well worthwhile to lose weight.

From the psychological and personal perspective, you ought to

*These opinions are summarized by Berger, M., Berchtold, P., Gries, A., and Zimmerman, H. 1981. Indications for the treatment of obesity. In P. Bjorntorp, M. Cairella, and A. N. Howard (eds.), *Recent Advances in Obesity Research: III.* London: John Libbey & Company Limited.

weigh whatever you want! *But* your desires must be tempered by several considerations.

The weight you desire should be consistent with your overall physical and mental health, and your emotional well-being is an important factor. It is ridiculous to live in a state of tension, dieting or exercising compulsively because you want to look like the fashion model on the cover of a woman's magazine, when *your* genes, operating through your hormones and enzymes, virtually dictate a bust, hips, or thighs that are fuller than average. Under these conditions, such behavior is harmful, physically and mentally.

Table A-1 presents the suggested weight ranges from the latest Build and Blood Pressure Study that related weight to longevity.* The weights in this table can be used as a rough guide, provided you are in good health and have no weight-related health problems. However, if you do, you should consult with your physician, if you haven't already done so, and determine whether losing some weight might be healthful, *or whether just getting active without making any special effort at weight loss* could not accomplish the same purpose. For example, elevated blood lipids, mild hypertension, and adult onset diabetes often respond to an active life-style without much if any weight loss.

The suggested weights in the table have caused a certain amount of controversy because they are, in general, several pounds higher than the desirable weights published in earlier tables. Critics, including many scientists and health organizations, point out that cigarette smokers, who tend to be both leaner than average and die somewhat younger, were left in the calculations. And other persons, who might be somewhat heavier than average and who also die younger, were *removed* from the calculations (persons with cardiovascular disease and diabetics). These latter persons were removed in the effort to present a clearer picture of the independent contribution of weight to the life span when disease is not present. But both these manipulations—leaving a group of lighter people known to die younger in the calculations and removing heavier people who tend to die younger—have the effect of elevating desirable weight in the table. In the opinion of many experts, this gives a misleading picture.

*Reproduced courtesy of the Metropolitan Life Insurance Company.

Finally, speaking once again from a psychological perspective, most persons start a weight-control program with a target weight in mind as well as a wished-for rate of loss—how many pounds per week they want to lose. Physicians as well as commercial weight-control programs seem to encourage this. As long as the target and the speed of approach are reasonable and reachable, the setting of such goals may do no harm. *But the only thing that is really under your control is your behavior, not the scale.* I'll return to this point in a moment.

If you are more than 10 or 15 pounds overweight, and have in the back of your mind a target weight that is *below* the top of the range in Table A-1, you may be setting yourself an unrealistic and possibly unhealthy goal. Let's find out through experience: I suggest that you set some subgoals, each consisting of a 10- to 15-pound loss, move on down, *see how you look and feel,* and then reevaluate. You may be ready for a "time-out" from any further immediate caloric restriction. Most people will lose this amount of weight in the first 28 days of the Metabolic Breakthrough Plan, and the Metabolic Breakthrough Activity Program will prevent regaining any weight. Or you may decide to continue with another block of 10 or 15 pounds' loss.

If you are still looking for that "20 pounds off in 14 days" or the "up to a pound a day" rate of loss that has attracted so many people to some very self-defeating diets—well, perhaps you are reading this book from back to front, or I have failed to get my points across. I suspect that nothing can be quite so discouraging in a weight management effort as starting with those expectations and failing to meet them, *or* actually meeting them and facing the speed with which the weight starts to come back on again the moment you stop dieting.

I am particularly concerned if, like millions of others in this country, your weight is already within the limits of Table A-1 and you are anxious to weigh less either for cosmetic reasons or because you think you will work, play, or feel better at a lower weight. *You are already within the range associated with good health and longevity.* Instead of focusing on losing weight, I think you will be happiest and healthiest if you simply start *behaving* in a more healthful manner— eating nutritiously and becoming more active. Let your body adapt to your healthful new behaviors. Looking and feeling better are

TABLE A-1

*Suggested Weights**

		MEN		
HEIGHT		SMALL	MEDIUM	LARGE
FEET	INCHES	FRAME	FRAME	FRAME
5	2	128–134	131–141	138–150
5	3	130–136	133–143	140–153
5	4	132–138	135–145	142–156
5	5	134–140	137–148	144–160
5	6	136–142	139–151	146–164
5	7	138–145	142–154	149–168
5	8	140–148	145–157	152–172
5	9	142–151	148–160	155–176
5	10	144–154	151–163	158–180
5	11	146–157	154–166	161–184
6	0	149–160	157–170	164–188
6	1	152–164	160–174	168–192
6	2	155–168	164–178	172–197
6	3	158–172	167–182	176–202
6	4	162–176	171–187	181–207

		WOMEN		
HEIGHT		SMALL	MEDIUM	LARGE
FEET	INCHES	FRAME	FRAME	FRAME
4	10	102–111	109–121	113–131
4	11	103–113	111–123	120–134
5	0	104–115	113–126	122–137
5	1	106–118	115–129	125–140
5	2	108–121	118–132	128–143
5	3	111–124	121–135	131–147
5	4	114–127	124–138	134–151
5	5	117–130	127–141	137–155
5	6	120–133	130–144	140–159
5	7	123–136	133–147	143–163
5	8	126–139	136–150	146–167
5	9	129–142	139–153	149–170
5	10	132–145	142–156	152–173
5	11	135–148	145–159	155–176
6	0	138–151	148–162	158–179

*Weights at ages 25–59 based on lowest mortality. Weight in pounds according to frame (in indoor clothing weighing 5 pounds for men and 3 pounds for women; shoes with 1-inch heels).

automatic consequences of a healthier life-style.

If you believe in setting a reasonable weight goal, and a reachable speed of weight loss will be helpful to you, naturally you should go ahead and do both of these things. But consider this: if those wishes require *behaviors* that you cannot sustain until you reach your goal and an impossible life-style thereafter, what will you have accomplished?

I'll end this book with the advice I give everyone who is about to enter one of my weight groups at Vanderbilt—focus your attention on the *behaviors* it will take to ensure permanent weight management, as well as on that target weight itself. The Nutrition Plan and Activity Program for both weight loss and maintenance that I have presented are not only healthful and workable, they're livable. They do not entail undue sacrifice, hardship, or discomfort—in fact, they make you feel good in addition to their payoff. So concentrate on setting up your life to make it easy to carry out the behaviors that lead to success. *Reachable, daily behavioral goals are the only way to assure the attainment of your long-term health, weight, and fitness goals.*

REFERENCES

CHAPTER 2

1. Bray, G. A. 1983. The energetics of obesity. *Medicine and Science in Sports and Exercise* 15(1): 32–40.
2. Garrow, J. S. 1978. *Energy balance and obesity in man.* New York: Elsevier/North-Holland Biomedical Press.
3. Bennett, W., and Gurin, J. 1982. *The dieter's dilemma: Eating less and weighing more.* New York: Basic Books.
4. Katahn, M., and McMinn, M. R. Obesity: A behavioral point of view. *Annals of the New York Academy of Science.* In press.
5. Sörbris, R., Nilsson-Ehle, P., Monti, M., and Wadsö, I. 1979. Differences in heat production between adipocytes from obese and normal weight individuals. *FEBS Letters* 101 (2): 411–14.

CHAPTER 3

1. Flatt, J.-P. 1980. Energetics of intermediary metabolism. In Ross Conference Report No. 1., *Assessment of Energy Metabolism in Health and Disease.* Columbus, OH: Ross Laboratories.
2. Apfelbaum, M. 1975. Influence of level of energy intake on energy expenditure in man: Effects of spontaneous intake, experimental starvation, and experimental overeating. In G. A. Bray (ed.), *Obesity in perspective.* Washington, D.C.: U.S. Department of Health, Education and Welfare.
3. Wooley, S. C., Wooley, D. W., and Dyrenforth, S. R. 1979. Theoretical, practical, and social issues in behavioral treatments of obesity. *Journal of Applied Behavior Analysis* 12:3–25.
4. Benedict, F. G., Miles, W. R., Roth, P., and Smith, M. 1919. *Human Vitality and Efficiency under Prolonged Restricted Diet.* Washington, D.C.: Carnegie Institute of Washington, Publication 280 (quoted from Gar-

row, J. S. 1978. *Energy balance and obesity in man.* New York: Elsevier/-North-Holland Biomedical Press, p. 89). This study is discussed in greater detail in Chapter 20.

5. Schwartz, R. S., and Brunzell, J. D. 1981. Adipose tissue lipoprotein lipase and obesity. In P. Björntorp, M. Cairella, and A. N. Howard (eds.), *Recent Advances in Obesity Research: III.* London: John Libbey & Company Limited.

6. DiGirolamo, M., Smith, U., and Björntorp, P. 1981. Refeeding effects on adipocyte metabolism. In P. Björntorp, M. Cairella, and A. N. Howard (eds.), *Recent Advances in Obesity Research: III.* London: John Libbey & Company Limited.

CHAPTER 4

1. Thompson, J. K., Jarvie, G. J., Lahey, B. B., and Cureton, K. J. 1982. Exercise and obesity: Etiology, physiology, and intervention. *Psychological Bulletin* 91:55–79.

2. Hollifield, G., and Parson, W. 1962. Metabolic adaptations to a "stuff and starve" feeding program. II. Obesity and the persistence of adaptive changes in adipose tissue and liver occurring in rats limited to a short daily feeding period. *Journal of Clinical Investigation* 41(2):250–53.

3. Fábry, P. 1967. Metabolic consequences of the pattern of food intake. In C. F. Code (ed.), *Handbook of Physiology,* Section 6, Volume 1, 31–50. Washington, D.C.: American Physiological Society.

4. Bray, G. A. 1983. The energetics of obesity. *Medicine and Science in Sports and Exercise* 15(1):32–40.

5. Flatt, J.-P. 1980. Energetics of intermediary metabolism. In Ross Conference Report No. 1., *Assessment of Energy Metabolism in Health and Disease.* Columbus, OH: Ross Laboratories.

CHAPTER 6

1. Vahouny, G. V. 1982. Conclusions and recommendations of the symposium on "Dietary Fibers in Health and Disease," Washington, D. C., 1981. *The American Journal of Clinical Nutrition* 35:152–56.

CHAPTER 7

1. Hensel, H., and Hildebrandt, G. 1964. Organ systems in adaptation: The muscular system. In D. B. Dill (ed.), *Handbook of Physiology,* Section 4, 73–90. Washington, D.C.: American Physiological Society.

2. Després, J. P., Bouchard, C., Savard, R., Marcotte, M., and Theriault, G. 1983. Effect of a twenty-week endurance training program on adipose tissue morphology and lipolysis in men and women. *Medicine and Science in Sports and Exercise* 15:138 (abstr.).

3. Leon, A. S., Conrad, J., Hunninghake, D. B., and Serfass, R. 1979.

Effects of a vigorous walking program on body composition and carbohydrate and lipid metabolism of obese young men. *American Journal of Clinical Nutrition* 32:1776–87.
4. Björntorp, P. 1983. Physiological and clinical aspects of exercise in obese persons. In R. L. Terjung (ed.), *Exercise and Sport Sciences Reviews.* Philadelphia: Franklin Institute Press.

CHAPTER 8

1. Katch, F. J., and McArdle, W. D. 1977. *Nutrition, weight control and exercise.* Boston: Houghton Mifflin.
2. Malina, R. M., Mueller, W. H., Bouchard, C., Shoup, R. F., and Lariviere, G. 1982. Fatness and fat patterning among athletes at the Montreal Olympic Games, 1976. *Medicine and Science in Sports and Exercise* 14(6):445–52.

CHAPTER 9

1. De Castro, J. M. 1978. Diurnal rhythms of behavioral effects on core temperature. *Physiology & Behavior* 21:883–86.
2. Zahorska-Markiewicz, B. 1980. Effects of timing on energy expenditure during rest and exercise in obese women. *Nutrition Metabolism* 29:238–43.
3. Koeslag, J. H. 1982. Post-exercise ketosis and the hormone response to exercise. *Medicine and Science in Sports and Exercise* 14(5):327–34.
4. Wilmore, J. H. 1983. Body composition in sport and exercise: Directions for future research. *Medicine and Science in Sports and Exercise* 15(1):21–31.
5. Miller, D. S., Mumford, P., and Stock, M. J. 1967. Gluttony. 2. Thermogenesis in overeating man. *The American Journal of Clinical Nutrition* 20:1223–29.
6. Zahorska-Markiewicz, B. 1980. Thermic effect of food and exercise in obesity. *European Journal of Applied Physiology* 44:231–35.

CHAPTER 10

1. Blair, S. N., Ellsworth, N. M., Haskell, W. L., Stern, M. P., Farquhar, J. W., and Wood, P. D. 1981. Comparison of nutrient intake in middle-aged men and women runners and controls. *Medicine and Science in Sports and Exercise* 13(5):310–15.
2. Katahn, M., Pleas, J., Thackery, M., and Wallston, K. A. 1982. Relationship of eating and activity self-reports to follow-up maintenance in the massively obese. *Behavior Therapy* 13:521–28.
3. Katahn, M., and McMinn, M. R. Obesity: A behavioral point of view. *Annals of the New York Academy of Science.* In press.

CHAPTER 12

1. Garrow, J. S. 1978. *Energy balance and obesity in man.* New York: Elsevier/North-Holland Biomedical Press.
2. Fisler, J. S., Drenick, E. J., Blumfield, D. E., and Swendseid, M. E. 1982. Nitrogen economy during very low calorie reducing diets: Quality and quantity of dietary protein. *The American Journal of Clinical Nutrition* 35:471–86.
3. Lantigua, R. A., Amatruda, J. M., Biddle, T. L., Forbes, G. B., and Lockwood, D. H. 1980. Cardiac arrythmias associated with a liquid protein diet for the treatment of obesity. *New England Journal of Medicine* 303:735–38.

CHAPTER 18

1. The material on which this chapter is based can be pursued in greater depth by consulting the following sources:
   (a) Jerome, N. W., Kandel, R. F., and Pelto, G. H. 1980. *Nutrional anthropology.* Pleasantville, NY: Redgrave Publishing Co.
   (b) Beller, A. S. 1977. *Fat and thin.* New York: Farrar, Staus, & Giroux.

CHAPTER 19

1. York, D. A. 1979. The characteristics of genetically obese mutants. In M. F. W. Festing (ed.), *Animal models of obesity.* New York: Oxford University Press.
2. Greenwood, M. R. C., Cleary, M., Steingrimsdottir, L., and Vasselli, J. R. 1981. Adipose tissue metabolism and genetic obesity: The LPL hypothesis. In P. Björntorp, M. Cairella, and A. N. Howard (eds.), *Recent Advances in Obesity Research: III.* London: John Libbey & Company Limited.
3. McCarthy, J. C. 1979. Normal variation in body fat and its inheritance. In M. F. W. Festing (ed.), *Animal models of obesity.* New York: Oxford University Press.
4. Bakwin, H. 1973. Body-weight reduction in twins. *Developmental Medicine and Child Neurology* 15:178–83.
5. Brook, C. G. D. 1977. Genetic aspects of obesity. *Postgraduate Medical Journal* 53:93–96.
6. Brook, C. G. D., Huntley, R. M. C., and Slack, J. 1975. Influence of heredity and environment in determination of skinfold thickness in children. *British Medical Journal* 2:719–21.
7. Borjeson, M. 1976. The aetiology of obesity in children. *Acta Paediatrica Scandinavica* 65:279–87.
8. Bennett, W., and Gurin, J. 1982. *The dieter's dilemma: Eating less and*

weighing more. New York: Basic Books.

9. Faust, I. M. 1981. Factors which affect adipocyte formation in the rat. In P. Björntorp, M. Cairella, and A. N. Howard (eds.), *Recent Advances in Obesity Research: III.* London: John Libbey & Company Limited.

10. Flatt, J.-P. 1980. Energetics of intermediary metabolism. In Ross Conference Report No. 1., *Assessment of Energy Metabolism in Health and Disease.* Columbus, OH: Ross Laboratories.

11. Glick, Z., Teague, R. J., and Bray G. A. 1981. Brown adipose tissue: Thermic response increased by a single low protein, high carbohydrate meal. *Science* 213:1125–27.

12. Sörbris, R., Nilsson-Ehle, P., Monti, M., and Wadsö, I. 1979. Differences in heat production between adipocytes from obese and normal weight individuals. *FEBS Letters* 101(2):411–14.

13. Jéquier, E. 1981. Thermogenic regulation in man. In G. Enzi, G. Crepaldi, G. Pozza, and A. E. Renold (eds.), *Obesity: Pathogenesis and treatment.* New York: Academic Press.

14. Guernsey, D. L., and Morishige, W. K. 1979. Na$^+$ pump activity and nuclear T$_3$ receptors in tissues of genetically obese *(ob/ob)* mice. *Metabolism* 28:629–33.

15. Lin, M. H., Romsos, D. R., Akera, T., and Leveille, G. A. 1981. Functional correlates of Na$^+$, K$^+$-ATPase in lean and obese *(ob/ob)* mice. *Metabolism* 30:431–38.

16. Lin, M. H., Vander Tuig, J. G., Romsos, D. R., Akera, T., and Leveille, G. A. 1980. Heat production and Na$^+$–K$^+$-ATPase enzyme units in lean and obese *(ob/ob)* mice. *American Journal of Physiology* 238:E193–99.

17. De Luise, M., Blackburn, G. L., and Flier, J. S. 1980. Reduced activity of the red-cell sodium-potassium pump in human obesity. *New England Journal of Medicine* 303:1017–22.

18. Bray, G. A., Kral, J. G., and Björntorp, P. 1981. Hepatic sodium potassium-dependent ATPase in obesity. *New England Journal of Medicine* 304:-1580–85.

19. Rothwell, N. J., and Stock, M. J. 1979. A role for brown adipose tissue in diet-induced thermogenesis. *Nature* 281:31–35.

20. Rothwell, N. J., and Stock, M. J. 1981. Hyperphagia, thermogenesis, and leanness. In P. Björntorp, M. Cairella, and A. N. Howard (eds.), *Recent Advances in Obesity Research: III.* London: John Libbey & Company Limited.

21. Rothwell, N. J., Stock, M. J., and Wyllie M. G. 1981. Na$^+$, K$^+$-ATPase activity and noradrenaline turnover in brown adipose tissue of rats exhibiting diet-induced thermogenesis. *Biochemical Pharmacology* 30:-1709–12.

22. Trayhurn, P., Thurlby, P. L., Woodward, C. J. H., and James, W. P. T.

1979. Thermoregulation in genetically obese rodents: The relationship to metabolic efficiency. In M. F. W. Festing (ed.), *Animal models of obesity*. New YOrk: Oxford University Press.

23. Gruen, R., Hietanen, F., and Greenwood, M. R. C. 1978. Increased adipose tissue lipoprotein lipase activity during the development of the genetically obese rat *(fa/fa)*. *Metabolism* 27:1955–66.

24. Taskinen, M.-R., and Nikkila, E. A. 1977. Effects of caloric restriction on lipid metabolism in man. *Atherosclerosis* 32:289–99.

25. Taskinen, M.-R., and Nikkila, E. A. 1981. Lipoprotein lipase of adipose tissue and skeletal muscle in human obesity: Response to glucose and semistarvation. *Metabolism* 30:810–17.

26. Schwartz, R. S., and Brunzell, J. D. 1981. Adipose tissue lipoprotein lipase and obesity. In P. Björntorp, M. Cairella, and A. N. Howard (eds.), *Recent Advances in Obesity Research: III*. London: John Libbey & Company Limited.

27. Horton, E. S., Danforth, E., Jr., and Sims, E. A. H. 1981. Metabolism in man: The Vermont studies. In G. Enzi, G. Crepaldi, G. Pozza, and A. E. Renold (eds.), *Obesity: Pathogenesis and treatment*. New York: Academic Press.

28. DiGirolamo, M., Smith, U., and Björntorp, P. 1981. Refeeding effects on adipocyte metabolism. In P. Björntorp, M. Cairella, and A. N. Howard (eds.), *Recent Advances in Obesity Research: III*. London: John Libbey & Company Limited.

29. James, W. P. T., Trayhurn, P., and Garlick, P. 1981. The metabolic basis of subnormal thermogenesis in obesity. In P. Björntorp, M. Cairella, and A. N. Howard (eds.), *Recent Advances in Obesity Research: III*. London: John Libbey & Company Limited.

30. Guthrie, H. A. 1979. *Introductory nutrition*. St. Louis, MO: C. V. Mosby.

31. Bray, G. A. 1969. Effect of caloric restriction on energy expenditure in obese patients. *The Lancet* 2:397–98.

32. Galton, D. J., and Bray, G. A. 1967. Metabolism of alpha-glycerol phosphate in human adipose tissue in obesity. *Journal of Clinical Endocrinology and Metabolism* 27:1573–80.

33. James, W. P. T., and Trayhurn, P. 1976. An integrated view of the metabolic and genetic basis for obesity. *The Lancet* 2:770–73.

34. Newsholme, E. A. 1980. A possible metabolic basis for the control of body weight. *New England Journal of Medicine* 302:400–405.

35. Miller, B. G., Otto, W. R., Grimble, R. F., York, D. A., and Taylor, T. G. 1979. The relationship between energy intake and protein turnover in lean and genetically obese *(ob/ob)* mice. *British Journal of Nutrition* 42:185–99.

CHAPTER 20

1. Horton, E. S., Danforth, E., Jr., and Sims, E. A. H. 1981. Metabolism in man: The Vermont studies. In G. Enzi, G. Crepaldi, G. Pozza, and A. E. Renold (eds.), *Obesity: Pathogenesis and treatment.* New York: Academic Press.
2. Flatt, J-P. 1980. Energetics of intermediary metabolism. In Ross Conference Report No. 1., *Assessment of Energy Metabolism in Health and Disease.* Columbus, OH: Ross Laboratories.
3. Apfelbaum, M. 1975. Influence of level of energy intake on energy expenditure in man: Effects of spontaneous intake, experimental starvation, and experimental overeating. In G. A. Bray (ed.), *Obesity in perspective.* Washington, D.C.: U.S. Department of Health, Education and Welfare.
4. Garrow, J. S. 1978. *Energy balance and obesity in man.* New York: Elsevier/North-Holland Biomedical Press.
5. Bray, G. A. 1983. The energetics of obesity. *Medicine and Science in Sports and Exercise* 15(1):32–40.
6. Neumann, R. O. 1902. Experimentelle Beiträge zur Lehre von dem täglichen Nahrungsbedarf des Menschen unter besonderer Berücksichtigung der notwendigen Eiweissmenge. *Arch. Hyg. (Berl.)* 45:1. (As discussed in Bennett, W., and Gurin, J. 1982. *The dieter's dilemma: Eating less and weighing more.* New York: Basic Books; Garrow, J. S. 1978. *Energy balance and obesity in man.* New York: Elsevier/North-Holland Biomedical Press.)
7. Sukhatme, P. V., and Margen, S. 1982. Autoregulatory homestatic nature of energy balance. *The American Journal of Clinical Nutrition* 35:-355–65.
8. Benedict, F. G., Miles, W. R., Roth, P., and Smith, M. 1919. *Human Vitality and Efficiency under Prolonged Restricted Diet.* Washington, D.C.: Carnegie Institute of Washington, Publication 280 (quoted from Garrow, J. S. 1978. *Energy balance and obesity in man.* New York: Elsevier/North-Holland Biomedical Press, p. 89.)
9. DiGirolamo, M., Smith, U., and Björntorp, p. 1981. Refeeding effects on adipocyte metabolism. In P. Björntorp, M. Cairella, and A. N. Howard (eds.), *Recent Advances in Obesity Research: III.* London: John Libbey & Company Limited.
10. Katahn, M., and McMinn, M. R. Obesity: A behavioral point of view. *Annals of the New York Academy of Science.* In press.
11. Sclafani, A., and Springer, D. 1976. Dietary obesity in adult rats: Similarities to hypothalamic and human obesity syndromes. *Physiology & Behavior* 17:461–71.
12. Katahn, M., and Meng, H. C. 1983. Effects of practice fasting and

cafeteria feeding on body weight and fat cell activity in rats. Paper delivered at the Satellite Conference on Energy Regulation, International Congress on Obesity, Stowe, Vermont.

13. Rolls, B. J., Rowe, E. A., and Turner, R. C. 1980. Persistent obesity in rats following a period of consumption of a mixed, high energy diet. *Journal of Physiology* 298:415–27.

14. An extensive, in-depth review of the material presented in Chapters 19 and 20 has just been prepared by one of my colleagues and myself. Copies are available on request:
McMinn, M. R., and Katahn, M. Energy expenditure in obesity. Submitted for publication.

CHAPTER 21

1. Bradley, P. J. 1982. Is obesity an advantageous adaptation? *International Journal of Obesity* 6:43–52.

2. Wilmore, J. H. 1983. Body composition in sport and exercise: Directions for future research. *Medicine and Science in Sports and Exercise* 15(1):-21–31.

3. Woo, R., Garrow, J. S., and Pi-Sunyer, F. X. 1982. Effect of exercise on spontaneous calorie intake in obesity. *The American Journal of Clinical Nutrition* 36:470–77.

4. Woo, R., Garrow, J. S., and Pi-Sunyer, F. X. 1982. Voluntary food intake during prolonged exercise in obese women. *The American Journal of Clinical Nutrition* 36:478–84.

CHAPTER 22

1. Katahn, M., and McMinn, M. R. Obesity: A behavioral point of view. *Annals of the New York Academy of Science.* In press.

2. Stifler, L. T. P., Kaplan, G. D., and Lindewall, D. The role of physical activity in a comprehensive weight control program. Submitted for publication.

CHAPTER 23

1. Balabanski, L. 1979. Diet and physical performance in the rehabilitation of obesity. *Bibliotheca Nutritionet Dieta* 27:33–44.

CHAPTER 24

1. Buccola, V. A., and Stone, W. J. 1975. Effects of jogging and cycling programs on physiological and personality variables in aged men. *Research Quarterly* 46:134–39.

2. Hartung, G. H., and Farge, E. J. 1977. Personality and physiological

traits in middle-aged runners and joggers. *Journal of Gerontology* 32:-541–48.

3. Ismail, A. H., and Trachtman, L. E. 1973. Jogging the imagination. *Psychology Today* 6:79–82.

INDEX